Examining the Relationship between Trauma and Addiction

Trauma, trauma-related disorders, substance use, and addictive disorders often co-occur, and frequently play a role in the problems and issues that social workers contend with in their practice with individuals, families, and communities. Research shows that there is a relationship between trauma-related symptoms and problematic use of substances and other addictive behaviors. Individuals who experience these co-occurring problems have better outcomes when their issues are addressed with integrated treatment approaches. Trauma-informed care and trauma-specific treatment are therefore important components of effective social work interventions.

This book examines various types of trauma, such as intergenerational trauma, adverse childhood events, childhood sexual abuse, and minority stress, amongst various populations and settings, including Native Americans, homeless youth, drug court participants, and LGB adolescents. It also explores the challenges in delivering trauma services in outpatient addiction treatment settings. Furthermore, it provides practical information on how to implement trauma-informed approaches in addiction treatment, and offers insights into the experience of a trauma survivor who is also recovering from a substance use disorder.

This book was originally published as a special issue of the *Journal of Social Work Practice in the Addictions.*

Shelly A. Wiechelt is Associate Professor in the School of Social Work at the University of Maryland, Baltimore County, USA. She specializes in research and practice on trauma and addiction. She is an Associate Editor for the *Journal of Substance Use & Misuse.*

Shulamith Lala A. Straussner is Professor and Chair of the Practice Area, and Director of the Post-Master's Certificate Program in the Addictions at the Silver School of Social Work, New York University, USA. She is the founding Editor of the *Journal of Social Work Practice in the Addictions.*

Examining the Relationship between Trauma and Addiction

Edited by

Shelly A. Wiechelt and
Shulamith Lala A. Straussner

Routledge
Taylor & Francis Group
LONDON AND NEW YORK

First published 2016
by Routledge
2 Park Square, Milton Park, Abingdon, Oxon, OX14 4RN, UK

and by Routledge
711 Third Avenue, New York, NY 10017, USA

First issued in paperback 2017

Routledge is an imprint of the Taylor & Francis Group, an informa business

British Library Cataloguing in Publication Data
A catalogue record for this book is available from the British Library

ISBN 13: 978-1-138-10672-7 (pbk)
ISBN 13: 978-1-138-93708-6 (hbk)

Typeset in Garamond
by RefineCatch Limited, Bungay, Suffolk

Publisher's Note
The publisher accepts responsibility for any inconsistencies that may have arisen during the conversion of this book from journal articles to book chapters, namely the possible inclusion of journal terminology.

Contents

Citation Information vii
Notes on Contributors ix

1. Introduction: Examining the Relationship Between Trauma and Addiction 1
Shelly A. Wiechelt and Shulamith Lala A. Straussner

2. Intergenerational Trauma Among Substance-Using Native American, Latina, and White Mothers Living in the Southwestern United States 6
Sally Stevens, Rosi Andrade, Josephine Korchmaros, and Kelly Sharron

3. Adverse Childhood Experiences and Gambling: Results From a National Survey 25
Anjalee Sharma and Paul Sacco

4. The Effects of Childhood Sexual Abuse and Other Trauma on Drug Court Participants 44
Molly R. Wolf, Thomas H. Nochajski, and Hon. Mark G. Farrell

5. Factors Associated With Substance Use Disorders Among Traumatized Homeless Youth 66
Sanna J. Thompson, Kimberly Bender, Kristin M. Ferguson, and Yeonwoo Kim

6. Traumatic Experiences and Drug Use by LGB Adolescents: A Critical Review of Minority Stress 90
Jeremy Goldbach, Benjamin W. Fisher, and Shannon Dunlap

7. Factors Related to the Delivery of Trauma Services in Outpatient Treatment Programs 114
Joseph J. Shields, Peter J. Delany, and Kelley E. Smith

8. Trauma-Informed Care and Addiction Recovery: An Interview With Nancy J. Smyth, PhD, LCSW 130
Interview Conducted by Lori Holleran Steiker

9. A Place in the World 139
Kimberly D. Honaker

Index 143

Citation Information

The chapters in this book were originally published in the *Journal of Social Work Practice in the Addictions*, volume 15, issue 1 (January–March 2015). When citing this material, please use the original page numbering for each article, as follows:

Chapter 1

Introduction to the Special Issue: Examining the Relationship Between Trauma and Addiction
Shelly A. Wiechelt and Shulamith Lala A. Straussner
Journal of Social Work Practice in the Addictions, volume 15, issue 1 (January–March 2015) pp. 1–5

Chapter 2

Intergenerational Trauma Among Substance-Using Native American, Latina, and White Mothers Living in the Southwestern United States
Sally Stevens, Rosi Andrade, Josephine Korchmaros, and Kelly Sharron
Journal of Social Work Practice in the Addictions, volume 15, issue 1 (January–March 2015) pp. 6–24

Chapter 3

Adverse Childhood Experiences and Gambling: Results From a National Survey
Anjalee Sharma and Paul Sacco
Journal of Social Work Practice in the Addictions, volume 15, issue 1 (January–March 2015) pp. 25–43

Chapter 4

The Effects of Childhood Sexual Abuse and Other Trauma on Drug Court Participants
Molly R. Wolf, Thomas H. Nochajski, and Hon. Mark G. Farrell
Journal of Social Work Practice in the Addictions, volume 15, issue 1 (January–March 2015) pp. 44–65

Chapter 5

Factors Associated With Substance Use Disorders Among Traumatized Homeless Youth
Sanna J. Thompson, Kimberly Bender, Kristin M. Ferguson, and Yeonwoo Kim
Journal of Social Work Practice in the Addictions, volume 15, issue 1 (January–March 2015) pp. 66–89

Chapter 6

Traumatic Experiences and Drug Use by LGB Adolescents: A Critical Review of Minority Stress
Jeremy Goldbach, Benjamin W. Fisher, and Shannon Dunlap
Journal of Social Work Practice in the Addictions, volume 15, issue 1 (January–March 2015) pp. 90–113

Chapter 7

Factors Related to the Delivery of Trauma Services in Outpatient Treatment Programs
Joseph J. Shields, Peter J. Delany, and Kelley E. Smith
Journal of Social Work Practice in the Addictions, volume 15, issue 1 (January–March 2015) pp. 114–129

Chapter 8

Trauma-Informed Care and Addiction Recovery: An Interview With Nancy J. Smyth, PhD, LCSW
Interview Conducted by Lori Holleran Steiker
Journal of Social Work Practice in the Addictions, volume 15, issue 1 (January–March 2015) pp. 134–142

Chapter 9

A Place in the World
Kimberly D. Honaker
Journal of Social Work Practice in the Addictions, volume 15, issue 1 (January–March 2015) pp. 143–145

Notes on Contributors

Rosi Andrade is a Research Professor in the Southwest Institute for Research on Women at the University of Arizona, Tucson, Arizona, USA.

Kimberly Bender is an Associate Professor in the School of Social Work at the University of Denver, Colorado, USA.

Peter J. Delany is Director of the Center for Behavioral Health Statistics and Quality, Substance Abuse and Mental Health Services Administration, Rockville, Maryland, USA.

Shannon Dunlap is a PhD student in the School of Public Affairs at UCLA, Los Angeles, California, USA.

Mark G. Farrell is a Retired Senior Justice in the Amherst Therapeutic Drug Court, Amherst, New York, USA.

Kristin M. Ferguson is an Associate Professor in the Silberman School of Social Work at Hunter College, City University of New York, USA.

Benjamin W. Fisher is a PhD student at the Peabody Research Institute, Vanderbilt University, Nashville, Tennessee, USA.

Jeremy Goldbach is an Assistant Professor in the School of Social Work at the University of Southern California, Los Angeles, USA.

Kimberly D. Honaker is a Research Coordinator in Morgantown, West Virginia, USA.

Yeonwoo Kim is a PhD student in the School of Social Work at the University of Texas at Austin, Texas, USA.

Josephine Korchmaros is Director of Research Methods and Statistics in the Southwest Institute for Research on Women at the University of Arizona, Tucson, Arizona, USA.

Thomas H. Nochajski is a Research Professor in the School of Social Work at the University of Buffalo, New York, USA.

Paul Sacco is Assistant Professor in the School of Social Work at the University of Maryland, College Park, Maryland, USA.

Anjalee Sharma is a Research Assistant at the Friends Research Institute, Baltimore, Maryland, USA.

Kelly Sharron is a PhD student in the Department of Gender and Women's Studies at the University of Arizona, Tucson, Arizona, USA.

Joseph J. Shields is a Professor in the National Catholic School of Social Service at the Catholic University of America, Washington DC, USA.

Kelley E. Smith is a Project Director at the Center for Behavioral Health Statistics and Quality, Substance Abuse, and Mental Health Services Administration, Rockville, Maryland, USA.

Lori Holleran Steiker is an Associate Professor in the School of Social Work at the University of Texas at Austin, Texas, USA.

Sally Stevens is Executive Director and Professor in the Southwest Institute for Research on Women at the University of Arizona, Tucson, Arizona, USA.

Shulamith Lala A. Straussner is Professor and Chair of the Practice Area and Director of the Post-Master's Certificate Program in the Addictions at the Silver School of Social Work, New York University, USA.

Sanna J. Thompson is an Associate Professor in the School of Social Work at the University of Texas at Austin, Texas, USA.

Shelly A. Wiechelt is Associate Professor in the School of Social Work at the University of Maryland, Baltimore County, USA.

Molly R. Wolf is an Adjunct Assistant Professor in the Social Work Department of Edinboro University of Pennsylvania, Edinboro, Pennsylvania, USA.

Introduction: Examining the Relationship Between Trauma and Addiction

SHELLY A. WIECHELT, PhD
Associate Professor, School of Social Work, University of Maryland, Baltimore County, Baltimore, Maryland, USA

SHULAMITH LALA A. STRAUSSNER, DSW, LCSW
Professor, Silver School of Social Work, New York University, New York, New York, USA

Trauma and trauma-related disorders as well as substance misuse and substance use disorders are often integral to the problems and issues that social workers contend with in their practice. Furthermore, it is empirically well established that there is a link between trauma-related disorders and substance use disorders. Trauma-informed care is essential in the provision of effective services. Therefore, it is important for social workers to consider the intersection of trauma and substance misuse across service settings. The intersection of trauma and substance misuse is particularly salient for social workers who practice in behavioral health settings where mental health and substance use issues are primary concerns.

Exposure to traumatic stress is also associated with behavioral or "process" addictions. Process addictions such as sexual addiction and Internet gaming are frequently discussed in the clinical literature, but are not classified as mental disorders in the *Diagnostic and Statistical Manual of Mental Disorders* (5th ed. [*DSM–5*]; American Psychiatric Association, 2013). However, the *DSM–5* Task Force determined that there is sufficient empirical evidence to warrant including gambling in the substance-related and addictive disorders section of *DSM–5* (Straussner, 2013). Recognizing that social workers contend with process addictions in their practice, the *Journal of*

Social Work Practice in the Addictions is designed to include content on all addictive behaviors.

The purpose of this special issue is to provide social work researchers, educators, and practitioners with updated information on the intersection between trauma and addictive behavior. The preponderance of research regarding trauma and addictive behavior is in the area of substance misuse and the contents of this special issue reflect that. Despite our call for papers that included all addictive behaviors, the submissions we received were predominately about trauma and substance misuse. We are delighted that this issue does include an article that examines the relationship between exposure to traumatic stress and gambling.

Some background information is essential for the reader to consider the range of issues regarding trauma and substance use and misuse presented in this issue. Trauma is generally thought of as distressing events that are psychologically overwhelming for the individuals who experience them (Briere & Scott, 2006; Straussner & Calnan, 2014). The *DSM–5* (American Psychiatric Association, 2013) specifies what constitutes a traumatic event under criterion A for posttraumatic stress disorder (PTSD) and acute stress disorder: exposure to actual or threatened death, serious injury, or sexual violation via direct experience, witnessing in person, learning that a close friend or family member experienced such an event, or repeated extreme exposure to aversive details about traumatic events (not via electronic media, television, movies, or pictures unless work related).

Individuals' responses to traumatic stressors vary; some experience severe trauma reactions and develop PTSD, whereas others have very little reaction at all when exposed to the same event. A variety of factors such as pretrauma characteristics and experiences of the individual, the nature and severity of the traumatic event, individual perceptions, and posttrauma experiences interact and contribute to the development of a trauma reaction (Straussner & Calnan, 2014). In fact, most individuals experience a traumatic stressor in their lifetime (56%) and few (8%) develop PTSD (Kessler, Sonnega, Bromet, Hughes, & Nelson, 1995). Individuals who experience traumatic stressors might experience reactions that are chronic and pathological or delayed; they might experience symptoms and recover to preevent levels of functioning; or they might exhibit resilience and maintain stable and healthy functioning after being exposed to a potentially traumatic event (Bonanno, 2004). Individuals could experience acute stress disorder that remediates in a month, develop the more severe PTSD, or develop other disorders and symptoms such as depression, anxiety, dissociation, and substance use. Other trauma-related syndromes have been identified (complex PTSD, developmental trauma disorder, cultural, and historical trauma; see van der Kolk, 2005; Wiechelt, 2014; Wiechelt & Gryczynski, 2012) but not included as specific disorders in the *DSM–5*.

This special issue features six original articles on trauma and addiction-related topics, two reviews of important books on trauma, an informative dialogue with Dean Nancy Smyth about trauma-informed care, and Kimberly Honaker's moving narrative about her own experience with recovery from trauma and addiction.

The first article, "Intergenerational Trauma Among Substance-Using Native American, Latina, and White Mothers Living in the Southwestern United States," by Stevens and colleagues provides social workers with much needed insight into the historical and current life traumas that affect Native American women when compared to White and Latina women. This article is especially important because Native American women are an at-risk group for a range of traumatic experiences and have unique needs relative to their experience of historical trauma. The authors suggest micro-, mezzo-, and macro-level interventions to address trauma and substance use among Native American women that are both trauma-informed and culturally sensitive.

The second article, "Adverse Childhood Experiences and Gambling: Results from a National Survey," by Sharma and Sacco is a novel examination of childhood trauma and gambling. The findings from this study indicate that adverse events in childhood are associated with gambling problems among other mental health issues. Prevention and treatment efforts aimed at children and youth who have experienced adverse childhood events might reduce later risk for developing gambling problems.

The third article, "The Effects of Childhood Sexual Abuse and Other Trauma on Drug Court Participants," by Wolf, Nochajski, and Farrell, presents findings that suggest that drug courts should implement trauma-informed care. Drug courts are widely used in the United States in an effort to offer a rehabilitative rather than punitive option for addicted individuals. Drug court procedures and mandated treatment processes that are trauma-informed might result in higher success rates.

The fourth article, "Factors Associated With Substance Use Disorders Among Traumatized Homeless Youth," by Thompson and colleagues examines the effect of protective factors, homelessness lifestyle, and trauma-related risk factors on substance use among homeless youth. The findings indicate that interventions that promote protective factors such as increasing personal competency and social coping among homeless youth reduce the risk for substance use. This article is important because it provides new insight into the buffering effects of protective factors among homeless youth.

The fifth article, "Traumatic Experiences and Drug Use by LGB Adolescents: A Critical Review of Minority Stress," by Goldbach, Fisher, and Dunlap is a systematic review of the literature with implications for effective substance use treatment for lesbian, gay, and bisexual (LGB) youth. The authors introduce the notion that effective practice with substance-using

LGB youth should incorporate interventions that address the complexity of minority stress rather than focusing in on single stressors alone.

The sixth and final article, "Factors Related to the Delivery of Trauma Services in Outpatient Treatment Programs," by Shields, Delany, and Smith examines the perplexing question of why we do not have more substance abuse treatment programs that offer trauma services in light of the clear relationship between trauma and substance use disorders. Interestingly, their findings from national survey data show that organizations that treat those at perceived greater risk for trauma (e.g., women and veterans) are more likely to provide trauma services in their programs. They also found that organizational characteristics heavily influence the adoption of trauma services. It seems that we still cling to the notion that abstinence must be attained before trauma work can begin and we fail to recognize the importance of integrated treatment where trauma and substance abuse are concerned.

The collection of articles presented in this special issue addresses the relationship between trauma and addiction in a range of settings and populations. The contents are by no means exhaustive, but do offer new insights for social work practice with regard to trauma and addiction. The need for trauma-informed care and trauma-specific interventions in substance user treatment and prevention programs is clear. The Special Topics dialogue between Steiker and Smyth provides insight into trauma-informed care as well as practical information on how to move toward providing trauma-informed care and how to get more training to become skilled at delivering trauma-specific interventions. Probably the piece that matters most in this issue is the powerful story that Honaker has the courage to share with us; it serves as a clear example of the power that trauma has in the lives of addicted individuals and a reminder that social workers can deliver interventions that heal the human heart.

REFERENCES

American Psychiatric Association. (2013). *Diagnostic and statistical manual of mental disorders* (5th ed.). Arlington, VA: Author.

Bonanno, G. A. (2004). Loss, trauma, and human resilience: Have we underestimated the human capacity to thrive after extremely aversive events? *American Psychologist*, *59*, 20–28.

Briere, J., & Scott, C. (2006). *Principles of trauma therapy: A guide to symptoms, evaluation, and treatment*. Thousand Oaks, CA: Sage.

Kessler, R. C., Sonnega, A., Bromet, E., Hughes, M., & Nelson, C. (1995). Posttraumatic stress disorder in the national comorbidity survey. *Archives of General Psychiatry*, *52*, 1048–1060.

Straussner, S. L. A. (2013). The DSM–5 diagnostic criteria: What's new? *Journal of Social Work Practice in the Addictions*, *13*, 448–453. doi:10.1080/1533256X.2013.840199

Straussner, S. L. A., & Calnan, A. J. (2014). Trauma through the life cycle: A review of current literature. *Clinical Social Work Journal*, *42*, 323–335. doi:10.1007/s10615-014-0496-z

van der Kolk, B. A. (2005). Developmental trauma disorder: Toward a rational diagnosis for children with complex trauma histories. *Psychiatric Annals*, *35*, 401–408.

Wiechelt, S. A. (2014). Intersections between trauma and substance misuse: Implications for trauma-informed care. In S. L. A. Straussner (Ed.), *Clinical work with substance-abusing clients* (3rd ed., pp. 179–201). New York, NY: Guilford.

Wiechelt, S. A., & Gryczynski, J. (2012). Cultural and historical trauma among Native Americans. In S. Ringel & J. R. Brandell (Eds.), *Trauma: Contemporary directions in theory, practice, and research* (pp. 191–222). Thousand Oaks, CA: Sage.

Intergenerational Trauma Among Substance-Using Native American, Latina, and White Mothers Living in the Southwestern United States

SALLY STEVENS, PhD
Executive Director and Professor, Southwest Institute for Research on Women, University of Arizona, Tucson, Arizona, USA

ROSI ANDRADE, PhD
Research Professor, Southwest Institute for Research on Women, University of Arizona, Tucson, Arizona, USA

JOSEPHINE KORCHMAROS, PhD
Director of Research Methods and Statistics, Southwest Institute for Research on Women, University of Arizona, Tucson, Arizona, USA

KELLY SHARRON, MA
PhD Student, Department of Gender and Women's Studies, University of Arizona, Tucson, Arizona, USA

The high rates of traumatic experiences reported by women who use alcohol and drugs have been documented in the literature. This study builds on the existing literature by examining the experiences of intergenerational family loss trauma among 226 mothering female substance users from 3 racial and ethnic groups: Native American (26.5%), Latina (24.8%), and White (48.7%). Demographic information, substance use,

We wish to acknowledge and thank the women who participated in the HerStory to Health project. Their lives reveal a tenacity to survive their circumstances and through their participation they provided an opportunity for researchers and service providers to learn.

intergenerational exposure to mothering, and other family traumatic losses were compared across racial and ethnic groups. Data indicate both similarities and significant differences in demographic characteristics, type of drug use, and traumatic family loss experiences—with a higher percentage of Native American women reporting instances of intergenerational family loss. The extent of intergenerational family traumatic loss among women who use substances is discussed, along with social policies that perpetuate such loss. Recommendations for effectively intervening at the individual, family, and policy levels are presented.

Research in the field of addictions has illuminated the association between traumatic events and addictive disorders, calling for changes in approach at the structural level and implementation of effective interventions at the family and individual level. More recently, experts have called attention to different types of trauma including trauma experienced by individuals, trauma suffered historically by various groups over time, and trauma encountered within families across generations. Although this research has informed the field, there remains a wide gap in knowledge with regard to intergenerational trauma, particularly intergenerational mothering and other family loss trauma experienced by women from different racial and ethnic groups. To address this gap in knowledge, this article first offers an overview of different types of trauma followed by an examination of types and rates of intergenerational family loss among 226 Native American, Latina, and White substance-using women. Finally, based on findings from this study, we offer recommendations for addressing substance abuse and reducing intergenerational family loss trauma at the structural level as well as at the individual and family level for this population.

INDIVIDUAL, HISTORICAL, AND INTERGENERATIONAL TRAUMA

Several types of trauma have been discussed in the literature, including individual trauma, historical trauma, and intergenerational trauma (Stevens, Andrade, & Ruiz, 2009; Substance Abuse and Mental Health Services Administration [SAMHSA], 2014). Many people who use alcohol or illicit drugs experience trauma either as a child or an adult, including men and women from various racial and ethnic backgrounds (Powell, Stevens, Lo Dolce, Sinclair, & Swenson-Smith, 2012; Stevens et al., 2009; Whitesell, Beals, Mitchell, Manson, & Turner, 2009). The relationship between substance abuse and trauma is complex wherein substances might be used to cope with past experiences of trauma. Such use might then contribute to additional traumas given the contexts and settings in which substances are used, the impact of substance use on decision making, and effects of substance use on motor skills and functioning (Asberg & Renk, 2012; Stevens et al., 2009; Zinzow et al., 2010).

Defining trauma has been complicated. Diagnostic criteria for traumatic stress disorder have evolved with several iterations noted in the *Diagnostic and Statistical Manual of Mental Disorders* (*DSM*). The most recent 2013 version of the *DSM* now includes a category for trauma and stressor-related disorders across the life span. Individual-level trauma is characterized by a set of circumstances experienced by an individual as "physically or emotionally harmful or life threatening and that has lasting effects on the individual's functioning and mental, physical, social, emotional, or spiritual well-being" (SAMHSA, 2014, p. 7). With regard to individual trauma, a high percentage of substance-using women report instances of this type of trauma including childhood sexual abuse and rape (Stevens, 2012). Higher levels of sexual abuse severity during childhood and greater lifetime exposure to trauma have been associated with a higher rate of substance use (Ullman, Relyea, Peter-Hagene, & Vasquez, 2013). Thus, it is not surprising that research indicates that between 55% and 99% of women seeking substance abuse treatment also report experiences of physical abuse, sexual abuse, or both (Najavits, Weiss, & Shaw, 1997). In addition, individual trauma among substance-abusing women is associated with other negative consequences, including relationship difficulties and legal problems (Asberg & Renk, 2012), and risk for a wide range of lifetime mental health problems (Lanius, Vermetten, & Pain, 2010). Given this research, there has been a heightened focus on developing, facilitating, and researching trauma-informed interventions for working with women who have a substance use disorder (SUD) and childhood or adult experiences of individual trauma (Powell et al., 2012).

In addition to experiences of individual trauma, historical trauma has been identified as having an impact on one's self-worth and mental health, and is also thought to be associated with behaviors such as substance use, domestic violence, child abuse, and suicide (SAMHSA, 2014). Historical trauma, sometimes referred to as community trauma, is experienced by a group or community as a whole—whether it is a natural disaster or an infliction made by a person(s) on another group or community. Yellow Horse Brave Heart, Duran, and Duran (2012) defined historical trauma as the cumulative psychological wounding over the life span and across generations, emanating from massively experienced group trauma such as genocide. Experienced by many groups, and specifically Native Americans, historical trauma can manifest in (a) historical unresolved grief—grief resulting from a collectively experienced historical trauma that has not been acknowledged or resolved; (b) disenfranchised grief—a type of loss experienced when it cannot be expressed or mourned in public space; and (c) internalized oppression—which occurs when a group of people suffers from a sustained loss of power like the experience of genocide and ongoing disenfranchisement (Yellow Horse Brave Heart et al., 2012).

Intergenerational trauma refers to trauma that is manifested in psychological symptoms and is transferred to future generations (Yehuda, Halligan, & Bierer, 2001). Historical trauma that emanates from group or community trauma can be transmitted to future generations as can trauma experienced at the individual level. Intergenerational trauma experienced by the individual impacts the offspring of that person (Stevens, Andrade, Korchmaros, & Sharron, 2014). This psychological wounding impacts one's self-worth, mental health, and behaviors, and is passed from one generation to the next. Specifically, intergenerational family loss trauma has been shown to be associated with substance use problems (Kaplow, Saunders, Angold, & Costello, 2010).

Intergenerational traumatic family loss could be experienced (a) when a family member dies—particularly if the death is unexpected, or (b) through an ambiguous loss—which can occur when a family member is alive but unavailable—such as in the case of a missing person, when a mother is incarcerated, or when a child is removed from his or her family by child protective authorities. Ambiguous loss is more difficult to identify; unlike a family death, it is not as concrete or as final (Betz & Thorngren, 2006; Guidry, Simpson, Test, & Bloomfield, 2013).

The impact of intergenerational traumatic family loss through a death is documented in the literature. The death of a parent is consistently rated as one of the most stressful life events that a child or adolescent can experience (Melhem, Porta, Shamseddeen, Payne, & Brent, 2011) and is associated with a number of mental and behavioral health problems (Cohen & Mannarino, 2011; Kaplow et al., 2010; Melhem et al., 2011). Research on mothers who experience the unexpected death of a child is also associated with mental and behavioral health problems, including ambivalence about their own death and suicidal ideation (Harper, O'Connor, Dickson, & O'Carroll, 2011), and a heightened mortality in the first 2 years after the death of a child (Espinosa & Evans, 2013). Additionally, longitudinal research on bereaved parents indicates that they report more depressive symptoms, health problems, and marital disruption as well as poorer well-being 18 years following the death of a child when compared to parents who had not experienced a death of a child (Rogers, Floyd, Seltzer, Greenberg, & Hong, 2008).

Research on the impact of an ambiguous loss indicates negative effects on the child involved. Children of incarcerated parents might exhibit troubling behaviors, guilt and rage, and symptoms of posttraumatic stress disorder (Bockneck, Sanderson, & Britner, 2009). Parental incarceration is also associated with the likelihood of the child using illicit drugs (Roettger,

Swisher, Kuhl, & Chavez, 2011). Similarly, youth removed from their homes by child welfare officials experience ambiguous loss, with research indicating higher levels of mental health problems, pregnancies at a young age, and higher incarceration rates compared to peers not in foster care (Golonka, 2010). The negative impact on mothers who are separated from their children is also documented in the literature. Experiences of ambiguous loss are complex and not well understood, although powerlessness, self-worth, health problems, and substance use have been noted in the literature (Mayes & Llewellyn, 2012; Myhra, 2011; Nixon, Radtke, & Tutty, 2013).

GENDER AND RACE AND ETHNIC DISPARITIES

Gender disparities exist with regard to a number of health and well-being issues. Specifically related to this study, experiences of childhood abuse as well as adult abuse have been noted. For example, in a national sample of youth, girls had significantly higher odds of having experiences of penetrative sexual abuse (Maikovich-Fong & Jaffee, 2010). In a study on male and female adolescents in substance abuse treatment, findings indicated that girls had higher levels of traumatic stress compared to boys (Stevens, Murphy, & McKnight, 2003). In adult populations enrolled in substance abuse treatment, a higher percentage of women in report traumatic experiences including sexual and physical abuse (Stevens et al., 2009). Additionally, high levels of trauma exposure among women receiving child welfare services have been reported. Chemtob, Griffins, Tullberg, Rhoberts, and Ellis (2011) reported that 91.6% of mothers receiving child welfare services in New York City experienced at least one traumatic event and 92.2% reported that their children had been exposed to one or more traumas.

Racial and ethnic disparities have also been cited in the literature. Whereas national studies examine disparities by multiple race and ethnic groups, field research studies rarely focus on comparisons between Native American, Latina, and White populations. Disparities with regard to Native American women compared to other racial and ethnic groups have been highlighted in the literature including higher rates of illicit substance use, violence, poorer childbearing outcomes, and late entry into prenatal care (Palacios & Portillo, 2008). Specific to this study, disparities in substance use have been documented. Findings from 2007 to 2009 indicate that among women 18 years of age and older, 11.4% reported illicit drug use in the past year. Illicit drug use varied by race and ethnicity, with higher rates among non-Hispanic American Indian/Alaska Native (17.5%), compared to non-Hispanic White (11.9%) and Hispanic (9.4%) women. The report also noted that racial and ethnic differences for specific types of illicit drugs are similar to differences for any illicit drug use. However, rates of cocaine use were highest among non-Hispanic White (1.7%) and Hispanic (1.4%)

women (U.S. Health Resources and Services Administration, Maternal and Child Health Bureau, 2011).

Past research has also identified disparities between these racial and ethnic groups with regard to family loss. For example, the life expectancy for Native Americans in the United States is 5.2 years less than the overall average of all racial and ethnic groups combined (Evans-Campbell, 2008). In 2007, child mortality for Native American children ages 1 to 4 years was second highest (39.2 per 100,000). The child mortality rate was much lower for children 1 to 4 years of age for Latinos (25.2) and non-Latino Whites (25.8; Singh, 2010). Additionally, ethnic and racial disparities are evidenced in both the criminal justice and child welfare systems. Native Americans have been admitted to prison at over 4 times the rate of Whites, and Latinos at 2 times the rate of Whites. Native American females are admitted to prison at over 6 times the rate of White females (Hartney & Vuong, 2009). Racially and ethnically diverse families are disproportionally represented in the foster care system (Boyd, 2014; Foster, 2012). Native American and Alaskan Native children are 2.2 and Latino children are 0.9 times more likely to enter foster care as compared to White children (Summers, Wood, & Russell, 2012). The burden of intergenerational traumatic family loss, whether through an early death or through an ambiguous loss is thus disproportionately experienced by ethnic minority populations, particularly by Native Americans. How these larger data sets reflect the experiences of smaller subgroups is not well known—including the differential experiences of intergenerational traumatic family loss of substance using mothers across racial and ethnic groups.

RISK AND PROTECTIVE FACTORS OF INTERGENERATIONAL FAMILY LOSS

The framework of risk and protective factors has, in part, been established from longitudinal studies of people experiencing trauma and what factors contribute to delinquency, substance use, or violence; or the integration into society and healthy relationships. Risk and protective factors of family loss are not a result of a few dominant factors but rather multiple independent factors that include both personal dispositions and community and social support (Board, 2005). Various risks and protective factors coalesce with each contributing to or reducing the likelihood of a resilient outcome (Bonanno, Galea, Bucciarelli, & Vlahov, 2007). A number of individual-level factors have been shown to influence the outcome of a potentially traumatic event including demographic variations (e.g., males, older age, higher educated), social and emotional support, prior and current stress, favorable worldview, and capacity for positive emotion (Bonanno, Westphal, & Mancini, 2011).

The adoption of individual resilience to the level of the family emerged from family science and psychology (Patterson, 2002). Although the family often serves as an important protective factor for children's resilience to adversity or traumatic experiences, it can also serve as a risk factor (Hawley & DeHaan, 1996). Family resilience surfaces in the face of hardship and refers to qualities that enable a family to remain in equilibrium in times of adversity or trauma. Family resilience has a dynamic quality and is based on adaptation processes including access to resources and behavioral changes within the family that help them to make new meanings or worldviews (Patterson, 2002).

Within the resilience literature, cultural variations have been discussed with regard to the way in which trauma is interpreted as well as its effects on the individual (Buse, Burker, & Bernacchio, 2013), and specifically with regard to the handling of grief related to the death of a child (Doran & Nanson, 2006). For Native Americans, resilience may be increased, influenced by such factors as those related a heightened sense of spirituality and an emphasis on community over the individual (Hawley & DeHaan, 1996), as well as a close connections to one's cultural roots and engagement in rituals and ceremony (Buse et al., 2013). Within this literature, however, less attention has focused on race as a risk or protective factor, particularly among women of color who report substance abuse. In addition, much of the family resilience research has focused on familial coping with a child's trauma, rather than trauma experienced by a mother.

To further examine rates of intergenerational family loss experiences, including both death and ambiguous family loss, we analyzed data from 226 Native American, Latina, and White substance-using women enrolled in the HerStory to Health project. Because of the project's location in the U.S.–Mexico border region in Arizona, the majority of participants identified as Native American, Latina, or White, allowing for a unique comparison among these racial and ethnic groups with regard to substance use and intergenerational mothering and other family loss trauma. Given the literature on historical trauma and health disparities—specifically with regard to Native American women and children—as well as data that indicate disproportionate minority contact in the criminal justice and child welfare systems, we hypothesized that a higher percentage of Native American participants would report experiences of intergenerational traumatic family loss.

METHODS

This study analyzes data from the HerStory to Health project, a 6-year project (2008–2013) funded by SAMHSA. HerStory to Health provided a gender-specific comprehensive sexual health education program; HIV, STD, and Hepatitis B and C screening and treatment; trauma-informed treatment services—reflecting the intersection of trauma, substance use, mental health, and sexual risk behaviors in its approaches to services and treatment objectives; and recovery support activities. Participants included adult women recruited through (a) targeted street outreach to areas where homeless women are known to reside or obtain services, and (b) outreach at a local mother and child residential substance abuse treatment facility. The eligibility criteria for HerStory to Health included (a) being female, (b) being at least 18 years of age, and (c) having a past history of drugs or alcohol use. Those who met the entrance criteria completed the consent process and met individually and privately with project staff to complete the baseline assessment.

Baseline assessment data from a subgroup of HerStory to Health participants were used for this study. The inclusion criteria for this study included (a) providing valid data, defined as providing responses to at least 80% of the items on the baseline survey and not providing duplicate data (as some women participated in HerStory to Health multiple times); (b) identifying exclusively as Native American (identified as non-Latina and of American Indian race), Latina (identified as Latina and of White race or Latina and of no race), or White (identified as non-Latina and of White race); (c) having biological children under the age of 18. Of the 482 women enrolled in HerStory to Health, 39 did not provide valid data (25 were duplicate participants, 14 did not provide valid data that could be used to classify them as mothers or to categorize them by race or ethnicity); 83 were not exclusively Native American, Latina, or White; and 134 did not have any biological children under 18 years of age. Consequently, the final analytical sample is 226.

Assessment Measures

The measures included select measures from SAMHSA's Client Outcome Measures for Discretionary Programs Government Performance and Results Act (GPRA) Tool (http://www.samhsa-gpra.samhsa.gov) and the Comprehensive Assessment for Drug Involved Women (CADIW; Stevens, 2012; Stevens, Korchmaros, & Miller, 2010). The GPRA Tool assesses a variety of characteristics and behaviors such as drug and alcohol use and family and living conditions. The CADIW draws from several assessments that have been found to be acceptable, reliable, and valid for female substance-abusing populations. It assesses a variety of characteristics and behaviors such as drug and alcohol use and experiences with loss. The select measures utilized for this study are described in the following sections.

Demographic Measures

Demographic characteristics were assessed using items from the GPRA Tool and the CADIW. These included date of birth, level of education, marital status, employment, ethnicity, and race.

Substance Use

Primary drug of choice was assessed with one item from the CADIW. This item was open-ended and asked what is or was participants' primary drug of choice. On the GPRA Tool, participants were also asked if (yes or no) they had injected drugs during the past 30 days.

Exposure to Parental Difficulties as a Child

The CADIW included three questions on exposure to parental difficulties as a child. Participants reported whether (yes or no) they (a) had been abandoned by their parents, (b) had been a subject of a Child Protective Services (CPS) investigation, and (c) had been permanently removed from their home by CPS as a child.

Current Mothering Status

We define *mothering* as the social norms and legal parameters that allow a woman to care for and raise a child born to her without the intervention of the courts (i.e., severed parental rights) or a state-appointed body such as CPS. When these or other interventions curb mothering, women lose the social, cultural, or legal practice of mothering. The CADIW included items on current mothering. Participants reported how many children they gave birth to and the number of children, including nonbiological children, under the age of 18 currently in their care. Responses reflected the number of children birthed and currently in participants' care as reported by participants.

Participants also reported whether they had children living with someone else due to a child protection order. Those who answered in the affirmative were asked how many of their children were living with someone else due to a child protection order. Based on responses to these two questions, we created a variable that reflected the number of children living with someone else due to a child protection order, which ranged from zero (for those who did not have children living with someone else due to a child protection order) to six.

Family Loss

Multiple items included in the CADIW queried different types of family loss. Four of these items queried death of family members including death of their father, mother, partner, and child. Also asked about were three other types of family loss including whether participants had ever had a stillborn child, gone to jail or prison, and had a family member go to jail or prison. These items asked participants to respond with "yes" or "no."

RESULTS

Demographic Characteristics

Of the 226 participants, 60 were Native American (26.5%), 56 were Latina (24.8%), and 110 were White (48.7%). Of the Native American participants, 57.7% were from a tribe located relatively close to Tucson, Arizona, and 42.3% were from several other tribes located throughout Arizona. All Native Americans were urban dwellers with a few living in an urban area with back-and-forth mobility to their Native American reservation. Of the 226 participants, 62 (27%) were recruited through street outreach, with the remainder being recruited from the local mother and child residential substance abuse treatment facility. This percentage did not vary across racial or ethnic group ($\chi^2 = 2.39, p = .303$).

Comparisons of demographic characteristics, shown in Table 1, indicate disparities among Native American participants compared to Latina and White participants. Native Americans had disproportionately lower education levels as compared to Latinas and Whites (41.7% vs. 73.2% and 72.7% with at least a high school diploma, respectively). This difference is statistically significant, $p < .01$. In addition, Native Americans had disproportionately higher rates of unemployment (31.7% vs. 19.6% and 11.8% unemployed and looking for work) as compared to Latinas and Whites. This difference is also statistically significant, $p = .02$. Native American participants were also statistically significantly more likely than Latina and White participants to be single (70.0% vs. 55.3% and 50.9%).

Substance Use

As shown in Table 2, the results are similar to earlier studies of Native American women living in the same region with regard to self-reported high rates of alcohol use (Stevens, 2001). Native American participants were statistically significantly more likely to select alcohol (38.3% vs. 19.6% and 12.7%) and less likely to select methamphetamine (11.7% vs. 23.2% and 34.5%) as their primary drug of choice compared to Latina and White

TABLE 1 Demographic Information

Characteristic	Native American[a]	Latina[b]	White[c]	$\chi^2(df)$ Comparison $F(df)$	p
Average age	34.0	30.8	34.7	*3.68 (2, 23)	.03
% single or never married	70.0	55.3	50.9	9.01 (2)	.06
% high school graduate or higher	41.7	73.2	72.7	18.79 (2)	<.01
% unemployed and looking for work	31.7	19.6	11.8	12.39 (2)	.02

[a]$n = 60$, 26.5%. [b]$n = 56$, 24.8%, [c]$n = 110$, 48.7%.

TABLE 2 Primary Drug of Choice

Type of drug	Native American[a]	Latina[b]	White[c]	$\chi^2(2)$	p
Alcohol	38.3	19.6	12.7	6.33	.04
THC	13.3	16.1	12.7	0.53	.77
Cocaine	8.3	7.1	1.8	4.05	.12
Crack	13.3	7.1	3.6	4.73	.09
Heroin	1.7	7.1	8.2	3.46	.18
Methamphetamine	11.7	23.2	34.5	14.09	<.01
Unreported	15.0	23.2	25.5	2.51	.28
Ever injected drugs	21.7	17.9	39.1	10.34	.01

[a]$n = 60$. [b]$n = 56$. [c]$n = 110$.

participants. Furthermore, although not statistically significant, there was a trend for Native Americans to be less likely to select heroin as their primary drug of choice when compared to Latinas and Whites (1.7% vs. 7.1% and 8.2%). Additionally, White participants were significantly more likely to report having injected drugs (39.1%) compared to Native American and Latina participants (21.7% and 17.9%, respectively).

Exposure to Parental Difficulties as a Child

All racial and ethnic groups were exposed to parental difficulties as a child. The Native American, Latina, and White participants had similarly substantial proportions who were abandoned by their parents (41.7%, 44.6%, and 33.6%, respectively) with the highest percentage among Latinas. In addition, the groups reported somewhat similar rates of being a subject of a CPS investigation as a child with the highest percentage among Native American participants (25.0%) compared to Latina and White participants (16.1% and 17.3%). Although not significantly different, a strong trend indicated that the largest percentage of participants who were removed from their home by CPS were Native Americans compared to Latinas and Whites (16.7% vs. 8.9% and 5.5%).

Current Mothering Status

The racial and ethnic groups differed in current mothering status. As shown in Table 3, Native American participants had, on average, birthed the most children ($M = 3.8$) compared to Latina and White participants ($M = 2.9$ vs. $M = 2.6$). Latina participants had, on average, the most children under age 18 in their care ($M = 1.3$) compared to Native America and White participants ($M = 1.9$ vs. $M = 0.6$), respectively. Although not statistically significant, there was a trend, on average, for Native American participants to have the most children living with someone else due to a child protection order ($M = 1.3$ vs. $M = 0.8$) compared to Latina and White participants.

TABLE 3 Mothering Data

Characteristic	Native American[a]	Latina[b]	White[c]	χ^2 comparison $F(df)$	p
Exposure to parental difficulties as a child					
% abandoned by parents	41.7	44.6	33.6	2.25 (2)	.33
% subject of CPS investigation as a child	25.0	16.1	17.3	1.93 (2)	.38
% permanently removed from home by CPS as a child	16.7	8.9	5.5	5.80 (2)	.06
Current mothering status					
No. of children gave birth to	3.8	2.9	2.6	13.06 (2, 223)	<.01
No. of children under age 18 in care	1.0	1.3	0.6	5.72 (2, 223)	<.01
No. of children living with someone else due to child protection order	1.3	1.0	0.8	2.92 (2, 223)	.06

Note: CPS = child protective services.
[a]$n = 60$, 26.5%. [b]$n = 56$, 24.8%, [c]$n = 110$, 48.7%.

TABLE 4 Family Loss: Percentage % of Each Group Exposed During Lifetime

Type of event	Native American[a]	Latina[b]	White[c]	$\chi^2(2)$	p
Father died	50.0	19.6	31.8	12.27	<.01
Mother died	28.3	12.5	19.1	4.64	.09
Partner died	28.3	7.1	12.7	9.66	.01
Child died	20.0	7.1	10.9	4.84	.09
Child stillborn	8.3	7.1	3.5	2.12	.35
Went to jail or prison	90.0	85.7	83.6	1.29	.52
Family member went to jail or prison	78.3	71.4	60.9	5.80	.55

[a]$n = 60$. [b]$n = 56$. [c]$n = 110$.

Family Loss

The racial and ethnic groups differed in experiences of family loss, with the Native American participants experiencing disproportionate amounts of loss. As shown in Table 4, statistically significantly more Native American participants experienced the death of their father (50.0% vs. 19.6% and 31.8%) and their partner (28.3% vs. 7.1% and 12.7%) than Latina and White participants. In addition, although not statistically significant, there was a trend for more Native American participants to have experienced the death of their mother (28.3% vs. 12.5% and 19.1%) and the death of a child (20.0% vs. 7.1% and 10.9%) as compared to Latina and White participants.

DISCUSSION

Overall, the data demonstrate that a substantial percentage of mothering women from all three racial and ethnic groups did not graduate from high school and a high percentage were unemployed and looking for work. Data comparing the three groups illuminate disparities: A higher number of Native American women were without a high school degree and were unemployed. Without a high school diploma, there are fewer opportunities for employment and subsequently financial capability to adequately support themselves and their children. Although reasons for such substantial disparities in education and employment remain unknown, one is reminded of the historical trauma associated with the experience of Native Americans in boarding schools and the disrupted mothering. Although this was experienced by earlier generations, the need for culturally competent educational pedagogy and relevant educational practices remains. Structural changes in educational practices that include alternative ways of learning, mentoring, vocational development, and scholarship opportunities might increase engagement of Native American women in the formal educational process, resulting in enhanced employment opportunities and promoting protective factors that contribute to individual (e.g., higher education) and family (e.g., access to resources) resilience.

At the individual level, treatment, social services, and educational programs need to provide opportunities for the development of vocational skills while giving particular consideration to nontraditional careers (e.g., often higher paying careers typically occupied by men) that might allow for heightened opportunities for employment. General equivalency diploma classes should be available on site. Many Native Americans, especially those who live in more rural areas, as well as women of all racial and ethnic groups in treatment or recovery from SUDs, frequently lack computer or Internet access. Having computer workstations and flash drives to store homework, resumes, and employment application information is critical. Moreover, strengths-based approaches, particularly for women with past experiences of trauma who might not believe in their self-worth are called for. A program of peer mentoring for critiquing each other's work and practicing job-interviewing skills can provide for skill development as well as social support. These strategies also might contribute to increasing resiliency at both the individual and family levels among this population.

Although a substantial percentage of participants from all three racial and ethnic groups reported experiences of intergenerational difficulties related to mothering, Native American women more frequently reported being the subject of a CPS investigation and being removed from their home. These data hold across generations with Native American mothers also having fewer of their own children in their care and a higher number removed from their care. Native American experiences associated with a history of colonization and removal are manifested in these data. Other types of family loss were also experienced by a significantly higher percentage of Native American women, including the death of a father, mother, partner, and child. Moreover, although not statistically significant, a higher number of Native American women went to jail or prison, as did their family members. Given these data, structural changes within CPS and the criminal justice system are called for. The Adoption and Safe Families Act (ASFA) of 1997 mandated that parental rights be terminated if a child has been in foster care for 15 of the most recent 22 months, and if the parent(s) has not met the court-ordered reunification requirement. The intent of ASFA was to speed up the court system and to put pressure on parents to increase child reunification. Unfortunately, in the same year, only 31% of parents needing substance abuse treatment were able to receive it (Child Welfare League of America, 1997). Today the unmet treatment needs of women with SUDs continue to be unacceptably high, hampering and undermining reunification efforts, and calling for reform in child welfare and health care access for substance abuse treatment. Needed structural changes in the criminal justice system include changes in policies and practices that disrupt mothering. In Arizona, women are sent to prison facilities that can be well over 200 miles from their children. Economic and practical issues hinder mother–child visitation, which contributes to intergenerational family loss trauma, essentially punishing not only the mother, but the child as well. Having a cohesive mother–child bond that includes connectedness, communication, and time together enhances resiliency for both the mother and the child.

At the individual level, targeted outreach to engage mothers in substance abuse treatment, along with gender-specific, trauma-informed, and culturally competent treatment is needed. The identification of the high percentage of intergenerational family loss among Native Americans in this study makes it apparent that traditional medicine and institutionalized health care settings are insufficient. A non-Western model of therapeutic work is necessary to address individual, historical, and intergenerational trauma and loss. Cultural women's healing centers would be well suited to provide culturally driven, trauma-informed care that includes community and social support. A cultural healing center for Native American women would emphasize a holistic approach in which wellness is not simply the absence of disease from one's body, but rather an integration of one's body, mind, spirit, and emotion. Activities, led by individuals sanctioned to facilitate cultural activities, might include traditional teachings, stories, and ceremonies that enhance cultural identity and access traditional spirituality for the healing process. Many of these activities (e.g., talking circle, sweat lodge) are common among tribes, whereas others are tribe or region-specific (see Rowen et al., 2014, for a synthesis of cultural interventions for indigenous populations to treat addictions). Although additional research needs to be conducted on the effectiveness of culturally driven interventions, they currently provide promise for healing from substance abuse and experiences of personal and intergenerational family loss trauma.

With regard to assisting mothers experiencing intergenerational traumatic family loss, there is a substantial body of literature on the grief and loss process for coping with the death of a family member. The early work of Elizabeth Kübler-Ross outlined the stages of healing from this type of loss and the work for addressing the death of a family member. However, less is known about ambiguous traumatic family loss and effective approaches for working with people experiencing this type of loss. The high percentage of women who experienced this type of loss across ethnic groups in our study calls for an increased focus on strategies, both structural and individual, to reduce this type of loss and for clinically addressing ambiguous loss. These therapies and programs can be aligned with cultural beliefs and healing practices relevant to Native American women such as the talking circle and sweat lodge to optimize benefits.

Limitations and Recommendations

Several study limitations are worth noting. The sample is nonrepresentative and thus might not be generalizable to Native American, Latina, and White women living in different regions of the country or whose life context is different from those participating in this study. The study is cross-sectional. Many of the variables were measured with only one item (vs. a scale), and all data were collected through self-report. Although confidentiality was stressed and the researchers were not associated with a treatment program or governmental agency, the responses might be under- or overreported based on the participant's perception or lack of comfort with the topics in question.

The HerStory to Health project was able to highlight the specific needs of this population and attempt to provide gender-specific and culturally competent care only at the individual level. The larger structural issues demonstrated in the demographic, intergenerational mothering, and traumatic family loss data were not able to be addressed. A larger scope is needed to address the specific structural barriers that continue to be problematic. Some issues that might be addressed through advocacy include border rights and immigration reform, child protection and family reunification policies, prison reform, alternatives to traditional child care, and motherhood advocacy. These issues disproportionately affect Native American women and specifically those living in the Southwest borderlands region.

As Native Americans face heightened risk of child removal, additional research should be facilitated on the effects of child removal on mother and child's health and well-being. More intervention research also needs to be done on the best ways to work in Native and borderland communities. Additional research also needs to be conducted on how to best target care to Native American women experiencing intergenerational traumatic family loss.

CONCLUSION

In terms of care provided, HerStory to Health provides a model for targeting this specific community. The identification of needs made it evident that traditional medicine and institutionalized health care settings are not sufficient. A non-Western model of therapeutic work is necessary to address historical trauma, violence, and loss that intersect with health needs, and specifically SUDs. The experiences of trauma must be addressed simultaneously with health care. Health care and treatment providers also need to be aware of the stigma involved in women, particularly Native American women, seeking care, especially for substance abuse, trauma, and other health-related needs such as sexually transmitted infections. Increased access to resources and an emphasis on the availability of confidential care is essential to increasing engagement of this population in treatment and care.

REFERENCES

Adoption and Safe Care Act (ASCA) of 1997, Pub. L. No 105-89.

Asberg, K., & Renk, K. (2012). Substance use coping as a mediator of the relationship between trauma symptoms and substance use consequences among incarcerated females with childhood sexual abuse histories. *Substance Use & Misuse*, *47*, 799–808.

Betz, G., & Thorngren, J. M. (2006). Ambiguous loss and the family grieving process. *The Family Journal: Counseling and Therapy for Couples and Families*, *14*, 359–365. doi:10.1177/1066480706290052

Board, Y. J. (2005). *Risk and protective factors*. London, UK: Youth Justice Board for England and Wales. Retrieved from www.yjb.gov.uk/publications/resources/downloads/rpf%20report.pdf

Bockneck, E. L., Sanderson, J., & Britner, P. A., IV. (2009). Ambiguous loss and posttraumatic stress in school-age children of prisoners. *Journal of Child and Family Studies*, *18*, 323–333.

Bonanno, G. A., Galea, S., Bucciarelli, A., & Vlahov, D. (2007). What predicts resilience after disaster? The role of demographics, resources, and life stress. *Journal of Consulting and Clinical Psychology*, *75*, 671–672.

Bonanno, G. A., Westphal, M., & Mancini, A. D. (2011). Resilience to loss and potential trauma. *Annual Review of Clinical Psychology*, *7*, 511–535.

Boyd, R. (2014). African American disproportionality and disparity in child welfare: Toward a comprehensive conceptual framework. *Children and Youth Services Review*, *37*, 15–27.

Buse, N. A., Burker, E. J., & Bernacchio, C. (2013). Cultural variation in resilience as a response to traumatic experiences. *Journal of Rehabilitation*, *79*, 15–23.

Chemtob, C. M., Griffins, S., Tullberg, E., Rhoberts, E., & Ellis, P. (2011). Screening for trauma exposure, and posttraumatic stress disorder and depression symptoms among mothers receiving child welfare preventive services. *Child Welfare*, *90*(6), 109–127.

Child Welfare League of America. (1997). *Alcohol and other drug survey of state child welfare agencies*. Retrieved from www.cwla.org/programs/bhd/1997stateaodsurvey.htm

Cohen, J. A., & Mannarino, A. P. (2011). Supporting children with traumatic grief: What educators need to know. *School Psychology International*, *32*, 117–131.

Doran, G., & Hanson. D. (2006). Constructions of Mexican American family grief after death of a child: An exploratory study. *Cultural Diversity and Ethnic Minority Psychology*, *12*, 199–211. doi:10.1037/1099-9809.12.2.199

Espinosa, J., & Evans, W. N. (2013). Maternal bereavement: The heightened mortality of mothers after the death of a child. *Economics & Human Biology,11*, 371–381.

Evans-Campbell, T. (2008). Historical trauma in American Indian/Native Alaska communities: A multilevel framework for exploring impacts on individuals, families, and communities. *Journal of Interpersonal Violence*, *23*, 316–338.

Foster, C. H. (2012). Race and child welfare policy: State-level variations in disproportionality. *Race and Social Problems*, *4*, 93–101.

Golonka, S. (2010). *How states can best support older youth in foster care*. Washington, DC: National Governor's Association Center for Best Practices.

Guidry, K., Simpson, C., Test, T., & Bloomfield, C. (2013). Ambiguous loss and its effects on children: Implications and interventions for school counselors. *Journal of School Counseling*, *11*(15), 1–19.

Harper, M., O'Connor, R., Dickson, A., & O'Carroll, R. (2011). Mothers continuing bonds and ambivalence to personal mortality after the death of their child—An interpretative phenomenological analysis. *Psychology, Health & Medicine*, *16*(2), 203–214.

Hartney, C., & Vuong, L. (2009). *Created equal: Racial and ethnic disparities in the US criminal justice system*. Oakland, CA: National Council on Crime and Delinquency.

Hawley, D. R., & DeHaan, L. (1996). Towards a definition of family resilience: Integrating life-span and family perspectives. *Journal of Family Process*, *35*, 283–298.

Kaplow, J. B., Saunders, J., Angold, A., & Costello, E. J. (2010). Psychiatric symptoms in bereaved versus nonbereaved youth and young adults: A longitudinal epidemiological study. *Journal of the American Academy of Child & Adolescent Psychiatry*, *49*, 1145–1154.

Lanius, R. A., Vermetten, E., & Pain, C. (2010). *The impact of early life trauma on health and disease: The hidden epidemic*. Boston, MA: Cambridge University Press.

Maikovich-Fong, A. K., & Jaffee, S. R. (2010). Sex differences in childhood sexual abuse characteristics and victims' emotional and behavioral problems: Findings from a national sample of youth. *Child Abuse and Neglect*, *34*, 429–437.

Mayes, R., & Llewellyn, G. (2012). Mothering differently: Narratives of mothers with intellectual disability whose children have been compulsorily removed. *Journal of Intellectual & Developmental Disability*, *37*, 121–130. doi:10.3109/13668250.2012.673574

Melhem, N. M., Porta, G., Shamseddeen, W., Payne, M. W., & Brent, D. A. (2011). Grief in children and adolescents bereaved by sudden parental death. *Archives of General Psychiatry*, *68*, 911–919.

Myhra, L. L. (2011). "It runs in the family": Intergenerational transmission of historical trauma among urban American Indians and Alaska Natives in culturally specific sobriety maintenance programs. *American Indian and Alaska Native Mental Health Research: The Journal of the National Center*, *18*(2), 17–40.

Najavits, L. M., Weiss, R., & Shaw, S. (1997). The link between substance abuse and posttraumatic stress disorder in women: A research review. *American Journal of the Addictions*, *6*, 237–283.

Nixon, K. L., Radtke, H. L., & Tutty, L. M. (2013). "Every day it takes a piece of you away": Experiences of grief and loss among abused mothers involved with child protective services. *Journal of Public Child Welfare*, *7*, 172–193. doi:10.1080/15548732.2012.715268

Palacios, J. F., & Portillo, C. J. (2008). Understanding Native American women's health: Historical legacies. *Journal of Transcultural Nursing*, *20*(1), 15–27. doi:10.1177/1043659608325844

Patterson, J. M. (2002). Integrating family resilience and family stress theory. *Journal of Marriage and Family*, *64*, 349–360.

Powell, C., Stevens, S., Lo Dolce, B., Sinclair, K. O., & Swenson-Smith, C. (2012). Outcomes of a trauma-informed Arizona family drug court. *Journal of Social Work Practice in the Addictions*, *12*, 219–241.

Roettger, M., Swisher, R., Kuhl, D., & Chavez, J. (2011). Paternal incarceration and trajectories of marijuana and other illegal drug use from adolescence into young adulthood: Evidence from longitudinal panels of males and females in the United States. *Addiction*, *106*(1), 121–132. doi:10.1111/j.1360-0443.2010.03110.x

Rogers, C. H., Floyd, F., Seltzer, M. M., Greenberg, J., & Hong, J. (2008). Long-term effects of the death of a child on parents' adjustment in midlife. *Journal of Family Studies*, *22*, 203–211.

Rowen, M., Poole, N., Shea, B., Gone, J. P., Mykota, D., Farag, M., . . . Dell, C. (2014). Cultural interventions to treat addictions in indigenous populations: Findings from a scoping study. *Substance Abuse Treatment, Prevention, and Policy*, *9*, 34. doi:10.1186/1747-597X-9-34

Singh, G. K. (2010). *Child mortality in the United States, 1935–2007: Large racial and socioeconomic disparities have persisted over time*. Rockville, MD: U.S. Department of Health and Human Services, Health Resources and Services Administration, Maternal and Child Health Bureau.

Stevens, S. J. (2001). American Indian women and health. *Journal of Prevention and Intervention in the Community*, *22*, 97–109.

Stevens, S. (2012). Meeting the substance abuse treatment needs of lesbian, bisexual, and transgender women: Implications from research to practice. *Substance Abuse and Rehabilitation*, *3*, 27–36.

Stevens, S., Andrade, R., Korchmaros, J., & Sharron, K. (2014, February). *Health, opportunity, mothering and family loss disparities experienced by substance using Native American women living in Southwestern United States*. Paper presented at the 17th annual American Association of Behavioral & Social Sciences Conference, Las Vegas, NV.

Stevens, S., Andrade, R. A. C., & Ruiz, B. S. (2009). Women and substance abuse: Gender, age and cultural considerations. *Journal of Ethnicity in Substance Abuse*, *8*, 341–358.

Stevens, S., Korchmaros, J., & Miller, D. (2010). A comparison of victimization and perpetration of intimate partner violence among drug abusing heterosexual and lesbian women. *Journal of Family Violence*, *25*, 639–649.

Stevens, S. J., Murphy, B. S., & McKnight, K. (2003). Traumatic stress and gender differences in relationship to substance abuse, mental health, physical health, and HIV risk behavior in a sample of adolescents enrolled in drug treatment. *Child Maltreatment*, *8*(1), 46–57.

Substance Abuse and Mental Health Services Administration. (2014). *Trauma-informed care in behavioral health services* (Treatment Improvement Protocol [TIP] Series 57, HHS Publication No. [SMA] 13-4801). Rockville, MD: Author.

Summers, A., Wood, S., & Russell, J. (2012). *Disproportionality rates for children of color in foster care*. Reno, NV: National Council of Juvenile and Family Court Judges.

Ullman, S. E., Relyea, M., Peter-Hagene, L., & Vasquez, A. L. (2013). Trauma histories, substance use coping, PTSD, and problem substance use among sexual assault victims. *Addictive Behaviors*, *38*, 2219–2223.

U.S. Department of Health and Human Services, Health Resources and Services Administration, Maternal and Child Health Bureau. (2011). *Women's health USA*. Rockville, MD: Author.

Whitesell, N. R., Beals, J., Mitchell, C., Manson, S., & Turner, R. J. (2009). Childhood exposure to adversity and risk of substance-use disorder in two American Indian populations: The mediational role of early substance-use initiation. *Journal of Studies on Alcohol and Drugs*, *70*, 971–981.

Yehuda, R., Halligan, S. L., & Bierer, L. M. (2001). Relationship of parental trauma exposure and PTSD to PTSD, depressive and anxiety disorders in offspring. *Journal of Psychiatric Research*, *35*, 261–270.

Yellow Horse Brave Heart, M., Duran, B., & Duran, E. (2012). This is Indian country. Retrieved from www.webpages.uidaho.edu/engl484jj/historical_trauma.htm

Zinzow, H. M., Resnick, H. S., Amstadter, A. B., McCauley, J. L., Ruggiero, K. J., & Kilpatrick, D. G. (2010). Drug-or alcohol-facilitated, incapacitated, and forcible rape in relationship to mental health among a national sample of women. *Journal of Interpersonal Violence*, *25*, 2217–2236.

Adverse Childhood Experiences and Gambling: Results From a National Survey

ANJALEE SHARMA, MSW, LGSW
Research Assistant, Friends Research Institute, Baltimore, Maryland, USA

PAUL SACCO, PhD, LCSW
Assistant Professor, School of Social Work, University of Maryland, Baltimore, Maryland, USA

Pathological gambling disorder and problem gambling are addictive disorders with severe consequences for individuals, families, and society. Knowledge about associations between childhood adverse experiences (i.e., physical, sexual, and emotional abuse) and gambling pathology in adulthood is limited. Using data from the National Epidemiologic Survey on Alcohol and Related Conditions (NESARC), associations between adverse childhood experiences and lifetime gambling status were tested. Strong bivariate associations between adverse childhood experiences and gambling status were found, which were attenuated with the inclusion of clinical covariates. Adverse childhood experiences might be related to pathological gambling in adulthood, but this relationship might not be gambling-specific.

Pathological gambling disorder (PGD) and problem gambling (PG), a subclinical manifestation of PGD (Toce-Gerstein, Gerstein, & Volberg, 2003), are serious public health concerns that affect between 0.2%- and 2.0% of the adult population in the United States (Petry, Stinson, & Grant, 2005). Recently recategorized in the *Diagnostic and Statistical Manual of Mental Disorders* (5th ed. [DSM–5]; American Psychiatric Association, 2013) as a substance-related and addictive disorder, PGD is characterized by the endorsement of at least four of nine criteria involving symptoms such as loss of control, preoccupation, chasing losses, concealment, and significant personal (i.e., relationship, job, education, etc.) losses as a result of gambling.

Consequently, PGD has a myriad of negative consequences for individuals, families, and communities. The seminal Gambling Impact and Behavior Study estimated the societal cost of PG and PGD to be $5 billion in the form of health care costs and productivity losses (Gerstein et al., 1999). For example, Thompson, Gazel, and Rickman (2012) found that economic costs include lost work time, unemployment, bad debt, theft, civil court costs, criminal justice system costs, and other costs, which totaled $8,681 and $15,994 per taxpayer, per problem gambler, in Wisconsin and Connecticut, respectively. Important correlates of PGD include divorce (Black, Shaw, McCormick, & Allen, 2012), job loss (Gerstein et al., 1999), and poor self-rated health (Black, Shaw, McCormick, & Allen, 2013).

In this study, we aim to extend research on adverse childhood experiences (ACEs) and gambling by testing associations between different types of ACE and PG or PGD, as well as analyze whether gambling-specific risk is present after adjusting for lifetime comorbid mental health and substance abuse disorders, and assessing multiple levels of gambling from nonproblem gambling to PG and PGD.

ADVERSE CHILDHOOD EXPERIENCES AND PATHOLOGICAL GAMBLING

Given the personal, social, and economic havoc associated with PGD and PG, understanding the developmental precursors of gambling pathology is a worthwhile endeavor as a means of developing effective prevention and policy initiatives. ACEs are one type of early life occurrence that can play a role in the later development of psychopathology in adolescence and adulthood. ACEs are defined by the Centers for Disease Control in two broad categories: acts of commission and acts of omission (National Center for Injury Prevention and Control, 2014). Physical, sexual, and psychological abuse can fall under the rubric of acts of commission, whereas different forms of neglect (e.g., failure to provide for the medical, physical, and emotional needs of a child) are acts of omission.

Recent studies suggest that the likelihood of experiencing abuse, neglect, and other ACEs is quite high. Data on confirmed child maltreatment reports have estimated that approximately one in eight children will experience some form of maltreatment by age 18 (Wildeman et al., 2014). Data from the Adverse Childhood Experiences study estimated the prevalence of psychological abuse at 11.1%, physical abuse at 10.8%, and sexual abuse at 22.0% (Felitti et al., 1998). Data from Wave 2 (2004–2005) of the National

Epidemiologic Survey on Alcoholism and Related Conditions (NESARC) identified rates of physical neglect at 15.8%, physical abuse at 14.9%, emotional abuse at 12.0%, sexual abuse at 10.1%, and emotional neglect at 7.9% (Fenton et al., 2013).

A large body of literature suggests that ACEs are associated with later adult psychopathology (Fenton et al., 2013; Keyes et al., 2012; McLaughlin et al., 2010). Keyes et al. (2012) identified associations between types of ACEs (physical abuse and neglect, emotional abuse and neglect, and sexual abuse) and latent constructs of internalizing (e.g., depression) and externalizing (e.g., substance use disorders) pathology. Harford, Yi, and Grant (2014) found retrospective associations between childhood maltreatment and lifetime suicide attempts and interpersonal aggression. These findings point to the potential that ACEs influence the development of broad psychopathological risk. Included in this general framework of broad risk, those who experience ACEs are at higher risk of externalizing disorders like substance use disorder and other addictions (Dube, Anda, Felitti, Edwards, & Croft, 2002; Dube et al., 2003; Felitti et al., 1998).

Although extensive research has explored the association between ACEs and the development of psychopathology and addictive disorders, there is a relative paucity of research focused on the relationship between ACEs and gambling pathology (i.e., PG and PGD). Much of the available research has been conducted with treatment samples (Kausch, Rugle, & Rowland, 2006; Petry & Steinberg, 2005), case-control studies (Black et al., 2012), and community samples (Felsher, Derevensky, & Gupta, 2010; Hodgins et al., 2010). Treatment samples show very high rates of reported ACEs. Using a continuous measure of childhood trauma exposure, Petry and Steinberg (2005) identified levels of childhood trauma exposure in the moderate to severe range as compared with the general population. In a study of participants in a Veteran's Administration gambling treatment program, 64.0% reported an emotional trauma, 40.5% reported a physical trauma, and 24.3% reported a sexual trauma; 91.5% of participants reported that the trauma occurred in childhood (Kausch et al., 2006).

In community studies, researchers have estimated rates of ACEs lower than in treatment samples, but have identified associations between gambling pathology and ACEs. Hodgins et al. (2010) studied ACEs and PGD in a community sample and found that 36.2% of respondents endorsed some type of abuse (physical, emotional, or sexual) or neglect (physical or emotional) in childhood. In this study, greater childhood maltreatment was associated with more frequent gambling and greater PG severity. Using a case-control design, Black and colleagues (2012) were able to compare rates of different types of ACEs between those with PGD and controls. Individuals with PGD have higher odds of emotional, verbal, and sexual abuse than controls. Overall, those with PGD were four times more likely than controls to have experienced some type of childhood abuse. Research by Felsher et al.

(2010) studied gambling risk as a function of maltreatment in a sample of young adults (ages 17–22). They identified an association between level of gambling severity (e.g., PG) and the experience of various forms of abuse and neglect including emotional, physical, and sexual abuse, and physical neglect.

Current theories of gambling addiction are consistent with research evidence suggesting ACEs are associated with PG and PGD later in life, including the pathways model (Blaszczynski & Nower, 2002) and Jacobs's general theory of addictions (Jacobs, 1986). According to the pathways model, there are three pathways that can lead to pathological gambling. Of these pathways, at least two have correlates with emotional vulnerabilities, childhood disturbances, and substance abuse (Blaszczynski & Nower, 2002). The three pathway groups that are proposed by the model help to highlight specific subgroups of gamblers manifesting in impulse control over their behavior. The specific groups are behaviorally conditioned problem gamblers, emotionally vulnerable problem gamblers, and antisocial, impulsivist problem gamblers. This has great implications for etiology as well as clinical treatment. In the pathways model, both emotionally vulnerable gamblers and antisocial impulsivist pathways arise in part from childhood disturbance. In the general theory of addictions, Jacobs (1986) surmised that feeling "inferior, unwanted, unneeded and/or generally rejected by parents or significant others" is a predisposing factor for addiction (p. 17). This experience, although not synonymous with ACEs, is, conceptually, highly related.

SHARED RISK FACTORS FOR ACES AND GAMBLING

Theory and a nascent body of research point to a relationship between ACEs and later PG and PGD. Nonetheless, relationships identified between ACEs and PG and PGD might be a result of shared sociodemographic and clinical risk factors. For instance, PG and PGD gamblers are more likely to be of younger age, male, African American, separated or divorced, and have lower education and income levels (Blanco, Hasin, Petry, Stinson, & Grant, 2006; Cunningham-Williams, Cottler, Compton, & Spitznagel, 1998; Gerstein et al., 1999; Petry, 2005; Welte, Barnes, Tidwell, & Hoffman, 2008). Correlates of ACEs are similar, although not consistently in the same direction. One form of ACE, child sexual abuse, is more common among women and those who are divorced, widowed, or separated (Pérez-Fuentes et al., 2013). Research suggests that females and African American youth are at greater cumulative risk of maltreatment (Wildeman et al., 2014) and more broadly defined ACE (Felitti et al., 1998; Harford et al., 2014).

In addition to shared demographic risk factors, PG or PGD and a history of ACE are both associated with a broad range of cooccurring mental health, substance abuse, and personality disorders. Epidemiological studies support the idea that PG and PGD is comorbid with a range of disorders including, but not limited to, substance abuse, personality disorders, mood disorders, and anxiety disorders (Cunningham-Williams et al., 1998; Petry et al., 2005; Pietrzak, Morasco, Blanco, Grant, & Petry, 2007; Sacco, Cunningham-Williams, Ostmann, & Spitznagel, 2008). Likewise, a large body of research has implicated ACEs in adult psychopathology inclusive of mood disorders, anxiety disorders, substance use disorders, and personality disorders (Afifi et al., 2008; Chapman, Dube, & Anda, 2007; Norman et al., 2012). In assessing the relationship between ACE and PG or PGD, research should consider the role of these shared sociodemographic and clinical correlates. Research by Keyes and colleagues (2012) suggests that ACEs in childhood, rather than leading to a specific risk, confer broad risk of both internalizing and externalizing pathology.

As mentioned before, we aim to extend research on ACEs and gambling by testing associations between different types of ACEs, including but not limited to physical abuse, sexual abuse, and emotional neglect, and PG or PGD. Further, we aim to analyze whether gambling-specific risk is present after adjusting for lifetime comorbid mental health and substance abuse disorders, as well as assessing multiple levels of gambling from nonproblem gambling to PG and PGD. In this manner, it is possible to assess the role of ACEs on a meaningful continuum of gambling behaviors.

METHOD

Sample

Data for this analysis were from Wave 1: 2001–2002 (Chen et al., 2006) and Wave 2: 2004–2005 (Chen, Yi, Dawson, Stinson, & Grant, 2010) of the NESARC conducted by the National Institute on Alcohol Abuse and Alcoholism (NIAAA) in cooperation with the U.S Census Bureau. The NESARC survey was a landmark, nationally representative survey designed to estimate the prevalence and comorbidities of substance abuse and mental health conditions over two waves of data collection.

Specially trained census workers conducted in-person computer-assisted interviews using the Alcohol Use Disorders and Associated Disabilities Interview Schedule (AUDADIS; Grant et al., 2003; Grant, Harford, Dawson, Chou, & Pickering, 1995). The NESARC survey employed a multistage stratified sample designed to be representative of the civilian, noninstitutionalized adult population in the United States in the year 2000. Sampling weights were created in NESARC to account for oversampling, to account for survey nonresponse, and to derive population-level estimates. Respondents were sampled from all 50 states and the District of Columbia and certain groups were oversampled (African Americans, Hispanics, and young adults aged 18–24 years old).

In Wave 1, the 43,093 respondents that participated were interviewed with an overall response rate of 81%. Participants were reinterviewed in Wave 2 with a response rate of 86.7% (n = 34,653) with a cumulative response rate of 70.2% (Chen et al., 2010). Data from Wave 1 and Wave 2 were merged for this analysis as gambling levels were measured at Wave 1 and ACEs were measured at Wave 2.

Measures

Gambling assessment

Fifteen items from Wave 1 assessed 10 *Diagnostic and Statistical Manual of Mental Disorders* (4th ed. [*DSM–IV*]; American Psychiatric Association, 1994) criteria for pathological gambling using the AUDADIS instrument (Grant et al., 2003). Each of the 15 items was asked regarding past year (i.e., in the past 12 months) and before past year (before the past 12 months) gambling problems. Based on work by Petry (2005), lifetime pathological gambling was recoded into four levels, zero to three. In this study, we define our levels as 0 = nongambler, 1 = nonproblem gambler, 2 = problem gambler, and 3 = pathological gambling disorder, parallel to Petry (2005). Nongamblers had not gambled more than five times in any year of their life and nonproblem gamblers endorsed less than two PGD criteria. Problem gamblers endorsed two to four *DSM–IV* gambling criteria and those endorsing greater than or equal to five criteria were classified as having PGD.

Adverse childhood experiences

Measures of ACEs were administered at Wave 2 of the NESARC using new AUDADIS modules developed specifically for the NESARC survey (Ruan et al., 2008). Question items in the AUDADIS were patterned on the Childhood Trauma Questionnaire (CTQ; Wyatt, 1985) and the Conflict Tactics Scale (CTS; Straus, 1979). Using this measure, we created the dichotomous measures of the following domains: physical abuse, sexual abuse, emotional abuse, physical neglect, and family violence based on the work of Harford et al. (2014). The physical abuse subscale included two items on the frequency of hitting and other violent behaviors by parents as well as leaving a visible mark (Ruan et al., 2008). Sexual abuse was assessed using four questions that asked about touching, fondling, and intercourse. The emotional abuse items included questions about being threatened by one's primary caregiver, being sworn at, or being threatened in any other way that would give one the impression that they were in danger of being physically hurt. Physical neglect was defined using five items: These questions dealt with hazardous chores, being left alone unsupervised, going without basic necessities, going without meals, and not getting medical treatment when it is necessary. The family violence subscale focused specifically on violence from an adult male directed at one's mother or female caregiver. Four questions asked about whether one's mother or other female caregiver was victimized by one's father or other adult male caregiver (including pushing, shoving or throwing, kicking, biting or hitting with something hard, hitting repeatedly, or threatening with a weapon).

Most items were coded 0 = *never*, 1 = *almost never*, 2 = *sometimes*, 3 = *often, and* 4 = *very often*. We recoded physical and emotional abuse as follows: If a respondent endorsed *often* or *very often* on any of the items in these subscales they were considered positive for that form of abuse. For sexual abuse, we used a lower benchmark based on work by Harford et al. (2014): If a person endorsed *almost never* or greater for any sexual abuse item, they were coded as having experienced sexual abuse.

Covariates

Model parameter estimates were adjusted using sociodemographic and clinical variables derived from Wave 1 of the NESARC survey. Self-identified gender was dummy coded (0/1) with male gender as one. We used a dummy-coded race variable using a five-level race and ethnicity (White, Black, American Indian/Alaskan Native, Asian/Pacific Islander, and Hispanic/Latino) variable constructed by the NESARC study team included in Wave 1. White race was used as the referent category. Age (18–29, 30–44, 45–64, 65+) and marital status (married, divorced, never married) were categorized into groups and dummy-coded. Education (less than high school, high school, some college or higher) and income (<$19,999, $20,000–$34,999, $35,000–$69,999, >$70,000) were also reorganized into groupings for analysis and dummy-coded. Using past-year and lifetime diagnostic variables in Wave 1, we created dichotomous variables for lifetime alcohol use disorder, drug use disorders (amphetamine, opioid, sedative, tranquilizer, cocaine, inhalant, hallucinogen, cannabis, heroin, and other), mood disorders (major depression, dysthymia, manic disorder, hypomanic disorder), anxiety disorders (panic disorder without agoraphobia, panic disorder with agoraphobia, agoraphobia, social phobia, specific phobia, generalized anxiety disorder). Using data from Wave 2, lifetime PTSD (occurring before measurement at Wave 1) was measured.

Data Analysis

Data analysis took place in two stages. First, we conducted bivariate analysis of sociodemographic covariates, ACEs, lifetime mental health disorders, and lifetime gambling levels (i.e., nongambler, nonproblem gambler, problem gambler, and pathological gambler). Following a descriptive analysis, multinomial logistic regression models were computed to assess relations between types of ACE and lifetime gambling status. To illustrate the impact of sociodemographic and clinical variables on these relationships, covariates were added to the models sequentially. First, bivariate models were estimated, and then sociodemographic variables were added to the models. Next, lifetime PTSD was added to the model followed by mood and anxiety disorders and finally substance use disorders. Odds ratios and 95% confidence intervals were calculated to illustrate the strength of relationships between these variables. All statistical modeling was conducted using SUDAAN 11® (Research Triangle Institute, 2012), software designed for analysis for complex survey data.

RESULTS

Sociodemographics, ACEs, Mental Health Disorders, and Gambling Status

Using bivariate models, we identified sociodemographic differences by gambling level (see Table 1). Males comprised only 43% of nongamblers, 58% of nonproblem gamblers, 67% of PGs, and 73% of PGD persons. African American respondents showed higher percentages of individuals in PG (16%) and PGD (21%) categories, as did Asian Americans (6% and 10%, respectively). Higher percentages of nongamblers (62%) and nonproblem gamblers (65%) were married, compared with lifetime PG (55%) and PGD (47%). Conversely, rates of being divorced or never married (17% and 25%) were slightly higher in the PG and PGD groups, respectively. Respondents aged 18 to 29 and 30 to 44 displayed higher levels of PG, and those aged 45 to 64 displayed higher percentages of PGD. Conversely, those over 65 were less likely to be in the PG and PGD groups. Those with less than a high school education were overrepresented in the PG and PGD groups and those with higher levels of education were less likely to be in the PG and PGD groups. In terms of income levels, those with the lowest income level ($0–$19,999) showed higher levels of PGD, and those with higher incomes ($35,000–$69,999 & $70,000+) were less likely to be in the PGD group

Table 2 displays bivariate associations between various forms of ACE and lifetime gambling status. The prevalence of every type of ACE was higher among PG and PGD groups with the exception of witnessing intimate partner violence (IPV) in childhood. In the nongamblers and nonproblem gamblers, rates of physical abuse were 4.40% and 4.84%, but among PGs and PGDs rates were 6.95% and 12.21%. Differences by gambling status were present for sexual abuse as well. Nongamblers (10.41%) and nonproblem gamblers (9.56%) displayed rates of sexual abuse of approximately 10%; among PG (15.50%) and PGD (15.44%) individuals, prevalence rates were more than 15%. Almost 20% of those with lifetime PGD reported emotional abuse, compared with approximately 8% in the nongambler and nonproblem

TABLE 1 Sociodemographic Covariates by Gambling Status

	NG[a]		NP[b]		PG[c]		PGD[d]		Wald	
	N	Wt. %	*n*	Wt. %	*n*	Wt. %	*n*	Wt. %	*F*	*p*
Male	9304	43.45	4,753	57.67	408	67.3	99	73.45	53.15	<.001
Race										
White	13,954	69.43	5,791	75.36	352	64.82	77	61.16	14.91	<.001
Black	4,656	11.04	1,696	10.49	172	15.73	53	21.30	7.85	<.001
AI/AN	383	2.01	176	2.57	18	3.84	3	1.23	2.84	.044
Asian/PI	726	4.59	208	3.27	25	5.85	7	9.94	6.56	<.001
Hispanic/Latino	4,994	12.90	1,240	8.30	106	9.77	16	6.38	9.83	<.001
Marital status										
Married	13,036	62.45	4,997	65.41	316	55.42	64	46.90	10.39	<.001
Divorced	5,999	16.08	2,357	17.32	157	17.10	51	24.84	3.07	.034
Never married	5,678	21.47	1,757	17.26	200	27.47	41	28.26	18.99	<.001
Age (in years)										
18–29	5,196	23.64	1,323	16.53	173	28.98	27	23.63	31.00	<.001
30–44	8,072	31.67	2,688	29.00	207	30.51	46	25.76	4.61	.006
45–64	7,209	28.75	3,405	36.84	230	32.01	73	43.20	26.90	<.001
65+	4,236	15.94	1,695	17.63	63	8.50	10	7.41	16.82	<.001
Education										
<High school	4,312	15.35	1,264	12.47	133	18.64	35	20.31	7.71	<.001
High school	6,105	24.91	2,358	26.19	194	29.12	31	22.59	2.71	.052
>High school	14,296	59.74	5,489	61.34	346	52.24	90	57.10	4.76	.005
Annual income										
$0–19,999	7,141	23.89	2,019	17.56	193	24.27	48	27.84	28.84	<.001
$20,000–34,999	5,225	29.84	1,949	19.93	142	19.94	36	22.18	0.09	.964
$35,000–69,999	7,537	32.08	3,102	35.32	215	33.34	45	31.38	6.19	<.001
$70,000+	4,810	24.19	2,041	27.18	123	22.45	27	18.61	5.33	.002

Note: NG = nongambler; NP = nonproblem gambler; PG = problem gambler; PGD = pathological gambler; AI/AN = American Indian/Alaskan Native; PI = Pacific Islander.
[a]n = 24,713. [b]n = 9,111. [c]n = 673. [d]n = 156.

TABLE 2 Adverse Childhood Experiences by Gambling Status

	NG[a]		NP[b]		PG[c]		PGD[d]		Wald	
	n	Wt. %	*n*	Wt. %	*N*	Wt. %	*n*	Wt. %	*F*	*p*
Physical abuse	1,194	4.40	479	4.84	58	6.95	23	12.21	3.81	.014
Sexual abuse	2,766	10.41	945	9.56	111	15.50	32	15.44	4.72	.005
Emotional abuse	1,996	7.52	787	8.20	97	11.61	31	19.06	5.93	.001
Physical neglect	2,019	7.39	756	8.03	76	10.18	32	17.73	3.61	.018
Witnessed IPV	904	3.27	342	3.33	45	4.95	10	5.19	1.31	.280

Note: NG = nongambler; NP = nonproblem gambler; PG = problem gambler; PGD = pathological gambler; IPV = intimate partner violence.
[a]n = 24,713. [b]n = 9,111. [c]n = 673. [d]n = 156.

gambler groups. Physical neglect was also more common among those in the PG and PGD categories, although the differences were less pronounced for PG. Physical neglect rates were between 7% and 8% for nongamblers and nonproblem gamblers, 10% for PG, and almost 18% for PGD.

TABLE 3 Lifetime Mental Health and Substance Use Disorders by Gambling Status

	NG[a]		NP[b]		PG[c]		PGD[d]		Wald	
	n	Wt. %	*N*	Wt. %	*N*	Wt. %	*n*	Wt. %	*F*	*p*
PTSD[e]	2,098	7.78	762	7.38	84	11.44	36	18.24	4.00	.013
Alcohol use disorder[f]	5,791	24.89	3,645	41.93	389	60.59	112	71.59	81.14	<.001
Drug use disorder[g]	2,031	8.86	1,148	12.68	190	29.92	51	36.55	34.61	<.001
Mood disorder[h]	5,203	20.38	2,022	20.81	300	43.58	96	54.54	23.74	<.001
Anxiety disorder[i]	4,206	16.63	1,790	19.17	249	38.64	75	42.70	22.24	<.001

Note: NG = nongambler; NP = nonproblem gambler; PG = problem gambler; PGD = pathological gambler; PTSD = posttraumatic stress disorder.
[a]*n* = 24,713. [b]*n* = 9,111. [c]*n* = 673. [d]*n* = 156. [e]PTSD assessed at Wave 2. [f]Alcohol abuse or dependence. [g]Amphetamine, sedative, tranquilizer, inhalant, hallucinogen, marijuana, or heroin disorder. [h]Major depressive disorder, dysthymia, or bipolar disorders. [i]Panic disorder, agoraphobia, social phobia, specific phobia, or generalized anxiety disorder.

We found similar differences by gambling status when assessing prevalence of lifetime gambling status and lifetime substance use and mental health disorders (Table 3). Each level of increased gambling pathology displayed higher prevalence of lifetime mental health disorder, although for some disorders, there was little difference between nongambler and nonproblem gambler groups. PTSD was more common in PG (11.44%) and PGD (18.24%) than in nongambler and nonproblem gambler groups (7.78% and 7.38%, respectively). Differences in lifetime alcohol use disorder by gambling disorder were monotonic, with 24.89% of nongambling respondents endorsing lifetime alcohol use disorder compared with 72.59% of those with PGD. We identified a similar pattern in lifetime drug use disorder, with the highest rates among those with lifetime PGD followed by progressively lower rates among lower levels of gambling involvement (i.e., PG, nonproblem gamblers, and nongamblers). For lifetime mood disorders, nongambler and nonproblem gambler rates were nearly the same at approximately 20%, but rates among those with PG (43.58%) and PGD (54.54%) were much higher. Anxiety disorders displayed a stair-step pattern (nongamblers, 16.63%; nonproblem gamblers, 19.17%; PG, 38.64%; and PGD, 42.70%) based on gambling status with the most pronounced differences within individuals with some form of problematic gambling.

Effects of ACEs on Risk of Gambling, Problem Gambling, and Pathological Gambling

Multinomial logistic regression models examined the association between ACEs and gambling disorders. Five models were estimated with the addition of statistical controls as follows: unadjusted; adjusted for sociodemographic covariates; adjusted for sociodemographic covariates and lifetime PTSD; adjusted for sociodemographic covariates, lifetime PTSD, and lifetime mood

TABLE 4 Multinomial Logistic Regression of Lifetime Gambling Status and Adverse Childhood Experience

	NP		PG		PGD	
	OR	95% CI	OR	95% CI	OR	95% CI
Unadjusted models						
Physical abuse	1.10	[0.97, 1.26]	1.62	[1.04, 2.53]*	3.02	[1.73, 5.29]**
Sexual abuse	0.91	[0.82, 1.01]	1.58	[1.18, 2.11]**	1.57	[0.96, 2.56]
Emotional abuse	1.10	[0.99, 1.22]	1.62	[1.23, 2.12]**	2.90	[1.67, 5.03]**
Physical neglect	1.10	[0.96, 1.24]	1.42	[0.99, 2.04]	2.70	[1.59, 4.60]**
Witnessed IPV	1.02	[0.88, 1.19]	1.54	[0.99, 2.39]	1.62	[0.79, 3.33]
Adjusted for sociodemographic variables[a]						
Physical abuse	1.16	[1.02, 1.32]*	1.62	[1.03, 2.55]*	2.96	[1.63, 5.35]**
Sexual abuse	1.07	[0.96, 1.18]	2.01	[1.48, 2.72]***	2.01	[1.22, 3.30]*
Emotional abuse	1.14	[1.02, 1.27]*	1.58	[1.19, 2.10]**	2.76	[1.54, 4.96]**
Physical neglect	1.14	[1.00, 1.30]*	1.44	[0.99, 2.09]	2.77	[1.65, 4.67]***
Witnessed IPV	1.18	[1.01, 1.39]*	1.69	[1.10, 2.59]*	1.81	[0.84, 3.94]
Adjusted for sociodemographic variables[a] and lifetime PTSD[b]						
Physical abuse	1.15	[1.01, 1.32]*	1.45	[0.89, 2.36]	2.36	[1.27, 4.38]**
Sexual abuse	1.06	[0.87, 1.17]	1.86	[1.33, 2.60]***	1.60	[0.98, 2.63]
Emotional abuse	1.13	[1.01, 1.26]*	1.44	[1.06, 1.96]*	2.27	[1.20, 4.30]*
Physical neglect	1.13	[1.00, 1.29]	1.31	[0.89, 1.94]	2.27	[1.30, 3.98]**
Witnessed IPV	1.18	[1.00, 1.38]	1.52	[0.99, 2.33]	1.41	[0.63, 3.16]
Adjusted for sociodemographic variables,[a] lifetime PTSD, and any lifetime mood/anxiety disorder[c]						
Physical abuse	1.12	[0.98, 1.28]	1.13	[0.69, 1.86]	1.78	[0.95, 3.34]
Sexual abuse	1.03	[0.93, 1.17]	1.42	[1.02, 1.98]*	1.18	[0.70, 1.98]
Emotional abuse	1.10	[0.98, 1.23]	1.13	[0.82, 1.54]	1.69	[0.88, 3.24]
Physical neglect	1.11	[0.98, 1.26]	1.07	[0.72, 1.59]	1.81	[1.04, 3.17]*
Witnessed IPV	1.15	[0.97, 1.35]	1.21	[0.78, 1.87]	1.06	[0.47, 2.40]
Adjusted for sociodemographic variables,[a] lifetime PTSD, mood/anxiety disorders,[c] and substance use disorder[d]						
Physical abuse	1.07	[0.93, 1.23]	0.97	[0.58, 1.60]	1.42	[0.76, 1.42]
Sexual abuse	0.99	[0.89, 1.10]	1.28	[0.92, 1.78]	1.00	[0.58, 1.70]
Emotional abuse	1.36	[0.71, 2.59]	0.95	[0.70, 1.30]	1.36	[0.71, 2.59]
Physical neglect	1.08	[0.95, 1.23]	0.99	[0.67, 1.47]	1.63	[0.93, 2.85]
Witnessed IPV	1.11	[0.94, 1.30]	1.09	[0.70, 1.70]	0.92	[0.39, 2.18]

Note: NG = nongambler; NP = nonproblem gambler; PG = problem gambler; PGD = pathological gambler; IPV = intimate partner violence; PTSD = posttraumatic stress disorder.
[a]Adjusted for demographics (sex, race, marital status, age, education, income). [b]PTSD assessed at Wave 2. [c]Panic disorder, agoraphobia, social phobia, specific phobia, generalized anxiety disorder, major depressive disorder, dysthymia, and bipolar disorders. [d]Alcohol use disorder, drug use disorder (amphetamine, sedative, tranquilizer, inhalant, hallucinogen, marijuana, and heroin).
*$p < .05$. **$p < .01$. ***$p < .001$.

or anxiety disorder; and adjusted for sociodemographics, PTSD, mood or anxiety disorder, and lifetime substance use disorder. Odds ratio estimates and 95% confidence intervals for models are reported in Table 4.

In unadjusted models we found that physical (OR = 1.62), sexual (OR = 1.58), and emotional abuse (OR = 1.62), were associated with approximately

60% greater odds of PG. Among individuals with physical abuse and neglect and emotional abuse, odds of PGD were nearly three times that of individuals who did not experience these forms of abuse.

Models adjusting for sociodemographic variables (Table 4) identified similar patterns of difference, with some exceptions. Those who experienced ACEs were slightly more likely to be nonproblem gamblers (with the exception of sexual abuse). Odds of PG were between 44% and 101% higher for all forms of ACEs, and odds of PGD were more than twice as high for those who experienced abuse and neglect. IPV was the only form of ACE not associated with PGD.

Inclusion of PTSD in statistical models narrowed risk somewhat. Individuals with a history of physical or emotional abuse were 13% and 15% more likely, respectively, to be nonproblem gamblers. Sexual abuse history was associated with 86% increased odds of PG, even after adjusting for comorbid lifetime PTSD. Similarly, emotional abuse was associated with 44% greater likelihood of lifetime PG. Odds of lifetime PGD were more than twice as high among individuals with physical and emotional abuse and physical neglect.

To assess gambling-specific risk because of ACEs, we estimated models that included lifetime mood and anxiety disorders and substance use disorders (Table 4). When adjusting for mood or anxiety disorders, sexual abuse was associated with 42% greater odds of PG, and physical neglect was associated with 81% greater odds of gambling. In the final model, we included lifetime alcohol and drug use disorders. When these disorders were included, associations between gambling level (e.g., nonproblem gambler) and ACEs were not statistically significant.

DISCUSSION

Our findings in a nationally representative sample add to an emerging body of evidence that ACE s are associated with gambling problems and pathological gambling (Black et al., 2012; Felsher et al., 2010; Hodgins et al., 2010; Petry & Steinberg, 2005). Although these associations do not appear to be a result of sociodemographic differences by gambling status, results of this analysis suggest that the risk of PG and PGD associated with ACEs are not gambling specific, but might reflect a generalized risk of adult mental health problems resulting from ACEs (Kessler et al., 2010; Keyes et al., 2012).

In this sense, problem and pathological gambling are one of many negative sequelae in adulthood arising from ACEs. Research findings suggest negative outcomes for psychological well-being and negative affect (Greenfield & Marks, 2010); alcohol dependence (Fenton et al., 2013); mood, anxiety, and substance use disorders (Afifi et al., 2008); smoking (Anda et al., 1999); and suicidality (Felitti et al., 1998; Harford et al., 2014; Pérez-Fuentes et al., 2013). ACEs such as maltreatment are precursors to a multitude of negative mental health outcomes in adulthood.

Multiple mechanisms might underlie the development of adulthood psychopathology, in general, and with PG and PGD in particular. From the perspective of neurobiology, a growing body of research suggests that ACEs have long-term negative structural and functional neurobiological correlates (McCrory, De Brito, & Viding, 2012) of ACEs (Anda et al., 2006) affecting areas such as executive functioning and emotion regulation (De Bellis & Zisk, 2014; Pechtel & Pizzagalli, 2011). Moreover, susceptibility to the effects of ACE on brain functioning could be moderated by levels of genetic risk.

Consistent with Jacobs's general theory of addiction and the pathways model, gambling behaviors might be a maladaptive means of regulating painful emotional states in a subpopulation of those with PGD who have experienced ACEs (Black et al., 2012; Blaszczynski & Nower, 2002; Jacobs, 1986). Research on endorsement of PG and PGD diagnostic criteria suggests that women in particular are more likely to endorse gambling to escape from their everyday problems (Sacco, Torres, Cunningham-Williams, Woods, & Unick, 2011).

ACEs could also cause deficits in executive functioning resulting from abuse and neglect. Studies conducted on the effects of child trauma on executive functioning suggest that these deficits are present in childhood (DePrince, Weinzierl, & Combs, 2009) and extend into adulthood (Gould et al., 2012; Nikulina & Widom, 2013). Consistent with the pathways model, the neurocognitive effects of ACEs are one mechanism in the development of pathological gambling through greater impulsivity and poor decision making.

Early family life factors such as a family history of PG or PGD might also influence both the likelihood of ACEs and the subsequent development of PG or PGD in adulthood (Black et al., 2014). Although ACEs were associated with PG and PGD in adulthood, it is notable that controlling for lifetime PTSD did not fully account for associations between ACEs and gambling. Potentially, problems with emotion regulation are generalized in individuals with ACEs and PTSD, and are not necessarily a function of maladaptive responses associated with PTSD symptoms.

Limitations

This study has a number of notable strengths including a nationally representative sample and the measurement of multiple levels of gambling involvement. Nonetheless, study findings should be interpreted in light of a number of limitations. NESARC survey respondents provided information on ACEs retrospectively, a method that might be less reliable due to recall bias. Further, research evidence suggests that retrospective reporting is associated with underreporting of abuse and neglect (Hardt & Rutter,

2004). Mental health and substance use disorders were measured as "lifetime," making the assessment of temporal associations impossible. Similarly, ACEs and PTSD were measured at Wave 2 of the NESARC and all other data were derived from Wave 1, potentially affecting the reliability of data and assessment of temporal relationships. Further, the sample size ($n = 156$) of pathological gamblers at Wave 2 limits the precision of standard errors, but nearly the same cell sizes have been used in other NESARC gambling analyses (see Petry et al., 2005). Finally, it is probable that unmeasured constructs (e.g., personality disorders, family history of gambling) could explain associations between ACEs and gambling, but were not assessed in this study.

From the standpoint of social work research, scholars in the field of child development and addictions might consider a longitudinal study of childhood maltreatment and PG or PGD using existing longitudinal data or child maltreatment data to disentangle the complex relationship of ACE and later substance abuse and mental illness problems, including PGD. We would advocate for the inclusion of gambling instruments in studies of human development.

Implications for Social Work Policy and Practice

Findings from this study provide a strong case for the valuable work of social work practitioners in child welfare. ACEs cast a long shadow into adult life in the form of mental illness and substance abuse. Our findings suggest that after controlling for demographic variables, the negative outcomes of ACEs are associated with PG and PGD. Social work practitioners and policymakers can play an important role in preventing ACEs and fostering the recovery of children and youth who experience maltreatment (Larkin, Felitti, & Anda, 2013). These efforts might help to decrease the prevalence of a variety of mental illnesses in adulthood, including gambling problems.

Because social workers commonly work with persons who experience multiple problems including a history of ACE, addictions, multiple psychiatric comorbidities, and family problems, they work extensively with individuals at high risk for gambling problems (Momper, 2010; Rogers, 2013). Therefore, practitioners would benefit from a more complete understanding of PGD assessment and intervention. A recent survey found that 38.4% of MSW programs include gambling-related content in their curriculum (Engel, Bechtold, Kim, & Mulvaney, 2012). Researchers advocated for greater inclusion of gambling assessment, treatment, and policy content in the MSW curriculum. Our study, although not specific to social work education, reinforces the importance of drawing connections between child protection and adult psychopathology for new practitioners with the understanding that their work reverberates into the future lives of the children they serve.

REFERENCES

Afifi, T. O., Enns, M. W., Cox, B. J., Asmundson, G. J. G., Stein, M. B., & Sareen, J. (2008). Population attributable fractions of psychiatric disorders and suicide ideation and attempts associated with adverse childhood experiences. *American Journal of Public Health, 98*, 946–952. doi:10.2105/AJPH.2007.120253

American Psychiatric Association. (1994). *Diagnostic and statistical manual of mental disorders* (4th ed.). Washington, DC: Author.

American Psychiatric Association. (2013). *Diagnostic and statistical manual of mental disorders* (5th ed.). Arlington, VA: Author.

Anda, R. F., Croft, J. B., Felitti, V. J., Nordenberg, D., Giles, W. H., Williamson, D. F., & Giovino, G. A. (1999). Adverse childhood experiences and smoking during adolescence and adulthood. *JAMA, 282*, 1652–1658.

Anda, R. F., Felitti, V. J., Bremner, J. D., Walker, J. D., Whitfield, C., Perry, B. D., . . . Giles, W. H. (2006). The enduring effects of abuse and related adverse experiences in childhood. A convergence of evidence from neurobiology and epidemiology. *European Archives of Psychiatry and Clinical Neuroscience, 256*, 174–186. doi:10.1007/s00406-005-0624-4

Black, D. W., Coryell, W. H., Crowe, R. R., McCormick, B., Shaw, M. C., & Allen, J. (2014). A direct, controlled, blind family study of DSM–IV pathological gambling. *The Journal of Clinical Psychiatry, 75*, 215–221. doi:10.4088/jcp.13m08566

Black, D. W., Shaw, M. C., McCormick, B. A., & Allen, J. (2012). Marital status, childhood maltreatment, and family dysfunction: A controlled study of pathological gambling. *Journal of Clinical Psychiatry, 73*, 1293–1297. doi:10.4088/JCP.12m07800

Black, D. W., Shaw, M., McCormick, B., & Allen, J. (2013). Pathological gambling: Relationship to obesity, self-reported chronic medical conditions, poor lifestyle choices, and impaired quality of life. *Comprehensive Psychiatry, 54*, 97–104. doi:10.1016/j.comppsych.2012.07.001

Blanco, C., Hasin, D. S., Petry, N., Stinson, F. S., & Grant, B. F. (2006). Sex differences in subclinical and DSM–IV pathological gambling: Results from the National Epidemiologic Survey on Alcohol and Related Conditions. *Psychological Medicine, 36*, 943–953. doi:10.1017/S0033291706007410

Blaszczynski, A., & Nower, L. (2002). A pathways model of problem and pathological gambling. *Addiction, 97*, 487–499. doi:10.1046/j.1360-0443.2002.00015.x

Chapman, D. P., Dube, S. R., & Anda, R. F. (2007). Adverse childhood events as risk factors for negative mental health outcomes. *Psychiatric Annals, 37*, 359–364.

Chen, C., Yi, H., Dawson, D., Stinson, F., & Grant, B. (2010). *Alcohol use and alcohol use disorders in the United States: A 3-year follow-up: Main findings from the 2004–2005 Wave 2 National Epidemiologic Survey on Alcohol and Related Conditions (NESARC)*. Bethesda, MD: National Institutes of Health.

Chen, C., Yi, H., Falk, D., Stinson, F., Dawson, D., & Grant, B. (2006). *Alcohol use and alcohol use disorders in the United States: Main findings from the 2001–2002 National Epidemiologic Survey on Alcohol and Related Conditions (NESARC)*. Bethesda, MD: National Institutes of Health.

Cunningham-Williams, R. M., Cottler, L. B., Compton, W. M., & Spitznagel, E. L. (1998). Taking chances: Problem gamblers and mental health disorders—Results from the St. Louis Epidemiological Catchment Area study. *American Journal of Public Health*, *88*, 1093–1096. doi:10.2105/AJPH.88.7.1093

De Bellis, M. D., & Zisk, A. (2014). The biological effects of childhood trauma. *Child and Adolescent Psychiatric Clinics of North America*, *23*, 185–222. doi:10.1016/j.chc.2014.01.002

DePrince, A. P., Weinzierl, K. M., & Combs, M. D. (2009). Executive function performance and trauma exposure in a community sample of children. *Child Abuse and Neglect*, *33*, 353–361. doi:http://dx.doi.org/10.1016/j.chiabu.2008.08.002

Dube, S. R., Anda, R. F., Felitti, V. J., Edwards, V. J., & Croft, J. B. (2002). Adverse childhood experiences and personal alcohol abuse as an adult. *Addictive Behaviors*, *27*, 713–725. doi:http://dx.doi.org/10.1016/S0306-4603(01)00204-0

Dube, S. R., Felitti, V. J., Dong, M., Chapman, D. P., Giles, W. H., & Anda, R. F. (2003). Childhood abuse, neglect, and household dysfunction and the risk of illicit drug use: The adverse childhood experiences study. *Pediatrics*, *111*, 564–572. doi:10.1542/peds.111.3.564

Engel, R. J., Bechtold, J., Kim, Y., & Mulvaney, E. (2012). Beating the odds: Preparing graduates to address gambling-related problems. *Journal of Social Work Education*, *48*, 321–335. doi:10.5175/JSWE.2012.201000128

Felitti, V. J., Anda, R. F., Nordenberg, D., Williamson, D. F., Spitz, A. M., Edwards, V., . . . Marks, J. S. (1998). Relationship of childhood abuse and household dysfunction to many of the leading causes of death in adults: The Adverse Childhood Experiences (ACE) Study. *American Journal of Preventive Medicine*, *14*, 245–258. doi:http://dx.doi.org/10.1016/S0749-3797(98)00017-8

Felsher, J. R., Derevensky, J. L., & Gupta, R. (2010). Young adults with gambling problems: The impact of childhood maltreatment. *International Journal of Mental Health and Addiction*, *8*, 545–556. doi:10.1007/s11469-009-9230-4

Fenton, M. C., Geier, T., Keyes, K., Skodol, A. E., Grant, B. F., & Hasin, D. S. (2013). Combined role of childhood maltreatment, family history, and gender in the risk for alcohol dependence. *Psychological Medicine*, *43*, 1045–1057. doi:10.1017/S0033291712001729

Gerstein, D., Hoffman, J., Larison, C., Engelman, L., Murphy, S., Palmer, A., . . . Hill, M. A. (1999). *Gambling impact and behavior study*. New York, NY: National Gambling Impact Study Commission.

Gould, F., Clarke, J., Heim, C., Harvey, P. D., Majer, M., & Nemeroff, C. B. (2012). The effects of child abuse and neglect on cognitive functioning in adulthood. *Journal of Psychiatric Research*, *46*, 500–506. doi:http://dx.doi.org/10.1016/j.jpsychires.2012.01.005

Grant, B. F., Dawson, D. A., Stinson, F. S., Chou, P. S., Kay, W., & Pickering, R. P. (2003). The Alcohol Use Disorder and Associated Interview Schedule–IV (AUDADIS–IV): Reliability of alcohol consumption, tobacco use, family history of depression and psychiatric diagnostic modules in a general population sample. *Drug and Alcohol Dependence*, *71*, 7–16. doi:10.1016/S0376-8716(03)00070-X

Grant, B. F., Harford, T. C., Dawson, D. A., Chou, P. S., & Pickering, R. P. (1995). The Alcohol Use Disorder and Associated Disabilities Interview Schedule

(AUDADIS): Reliability of alcohol and drug modules in a general population sample. *Drug and Alcohol Dependence*, *39*, 37–44. doi:10.1016/0376-8716(95)01134-K

Greenfield, E. A., & Marks, N. F. (2010). Identifying experiences of physical and psychological violence in childhood that jeopardize mental health in adulthood. *Child Abuse and Neglect*, *34*, 161–171. doi:S0145-2134(10)00040-2[pii]10.1016/j.chiabu.2009.08.012

Hardt, J., & Rutter, M. (2004). Validity of adult retrospective reports of adverse childhood experiences: review of the evidence. *Journal of Child Psychology and Psychiatry*, *45*, 260–273. doi:10.1111/j.1469-7610.2004.00218.x

Harford, T. C., Yi, H.-Y., & Grant, B. F. (2014). Associations between childhood abuse and interpersonal aggression and suicide attempt among U.S. adults in a national study. *Child Abuse and Neglect*, *38*, 1389–1398. doi:10.1016/j.chiabu.2014.02.011

Hodgins, D. C., Schopflocher, D. P., el-Guebaly, N., Casey, D. M., Smith, G. J., Williams, R. J., & Wood, R. T. (2010). The association between childhood maltreatment and gambling problems in a community sample of adult men and women. *Psychology of Addictive Behaviors*, *24*, 548–554. doi:10.1037/a0019946

Jacobs, D. F. (1986). A general theory of addictions: A new theoretical model. *Journal of Gambling Behavior*, *2*(1), 15–31.

Kausch, O., Rugle, L., & Rowland, D. Y. (2006). Lifetime histories of trauma among pathological gamblers. *American Journal on Addictions*, *15*(1), 35–43. doi:10.1080/10550490500419045

Kessler, R. C., McLaughlin, K. A., Green, J. G., Gruber, M. J., Sampson, N. A., Zaslavsky, A. M., . . . Williams, D. R. (2010). Childhood adversities and adult psychopathology in the WHO World Mental Health Surveys. *The British Journal of Psychiatry*, *197*, 378–385. doi:10.1192/bjp.bp.110.080499

Keyes, K. M., Eaton, N. R., Krueger, R. F., McLaughlin, K. A., Wall, M. M., Grant, B. F., & Hasin, D. S. (2012). Childhood maltreatment and the structure of common psychiatric disorders. *British Journal of Psychiatry*, *200*, 107–115. doi:10.1192/bjp.bp.111.093062

Larkin, H., Felitti, V. J., & Anda, R. F. (2013). Social work and adverse childhood experiences research: Implications for practice and health policy. *Social Work in Public Health*, *29*(1), 1–16. doi:10.1080/19371918.2011.619433

McCrory, E., De Brito, S. A., & Viding, E. (2012). The link between child abuse and psychopathology: A review of neurobiological and genetic research. *Journal of the Royal Society of Medicine*, *105*, 151–156. doi:10.1258/jrsm.2011.110222

McLaughlin, K. A., Green, J., Gruber, M. J., Sampson, N. A., Zaslavsky, A. M., & Kessler, R. C. (2010). Childhood adversities and adult psychiatric disorders in the National Comorbidity Survey Replication II Associations with persistence of DSM–IV disorders. *Archives of General Psychiatry*, *67*, 124–132. doi:10.1001/archgenpsychiatry.2009.187

Momper, S. L. (2010). Implications of American Indian gambling for social work research and practice. *Social Work*, *55*, 139–146. doi:10.1093/sw/55.2.139

National Center for Injury Prevention and Control. (2014). Child maltreatment: Definitions. Retrieved from http://www.cdc.gov/violenceprevention/childmaltreatment/definitions.html

Nikulina, V., & Widom, C. S. (2013). Child maltreatment and executive functioning in middle adulthood: A prospective examination. *Neuropsychology*, *27*, 417–427. doi:10.1037/a0032811

Norman, R. E., Byambaa, M., De, R., Butchart, A., Scott, J., & Vos, T. (2012). The long-term health consequences of child physical abuse, emotional abuse, and neglect: A systematic review and meta-analysis. *PLoS Medicine*, *9*(11), e1001349. doi:10.1371/journal.pmed.1001349

Pechtel, P., & Pizzagalli, D. (2011). Effects of early life stress on cognitive and affective function: An integrated review of human literature. *Psychopharmacology*, *214*, 55–70. doi:10.1007/s00213-010-2009-2

Pérez-Fuentes, G., Olfson, M., Villegas, L., Morcillo, C., Wang, S., & Blanco, C. (2013). Prevalence and correlates of child sexual abuse: A national study. *Comprehensive Psychiatry*, *54*(1), 16–27. doi:http://dx.doi.org/10.1016/j.comppsych.2012.05.010

Petry, N. M. (2005). *Pathological gambling: Etiology, comorbidity, and treatment*. Washington, DC: American Psychological Association.

Petry, N. M., & Steinberg, K. L. (2005). Childhood maltreatment in male and female treatment-seeking pathological gamblers. *Psychology of Addictive Behaviors*, *19*, 226–229. doi:10.1037/0893-164X.19.2.226

Petry, N. M., Stinson, F. S., & Grant, B. F. (2005). Comorbidity of DSM–IV pathological gambling and other psychiatric disorders: Results from the National Epidemiological Survey on Alcohol and Related Conditions. *Journal of Clinical Psychiatry*, *66*, 564–574. doi:10.4088/JCP.v66n0504

Pietrzak, R. H., Morasco, B. J., Blanco, C., Grant, B. F., & Petry, N. M. (2007). Gambling level and psychiatric and medical disorders in older adults: Results from the National Epidemiologic Survey on Alcohol and Related Conditions. *American Journal of Geriatric Psychiatry*, *15*, 301–313. doi:10.1097/01.JGP.0000239353.40880.cc

Research Triangle Institute. (2012). *SUDAAN Language manual, release 11*. Research Triangle Park, NC: Research Triangle Institute.

Rogers, J. (2013). Problem gambling: A suitable case for social work? *Practice*, *25*(1), 41–60. doi:10.1080/09503153.2013.775234

Ruan, W. J., Goldstein, R. B., Chou, S. P., Smith, S. M., Saha, T. D., Pickering, R. P., . . . Grant, B. F. (2008). The Alcohol Use Disorder and Associated Disabilities Interview Schedule–IV (AUDADIS–IV): Reliability of new psychiatric diagnostic modules and risk factors in a general population sample. *Drug and Alcohol Dependence*, *92*(1–3), 27–36. doi:10.1016/j.drugalcdep.2007.06.001

Sacco, P., Cunningham-Williams, R. M., Ostmann, E., & Spitznagel, E. L., Jr. (2008). The association between gambling pathology and personality disorders. *Journal of Psychiatric Research*, *42*, 1122–1130. doi:10.1016/j.jpsychires.2007.11.007

Sacco, P., Torres, L. R., Cunningham-Williams, R. M., Woods, C., & Unick, G. J. (2011). Differential item functioning of pathological gambling criteria: An examination of gender, race/ethnicity, and age. *Journal of Gambling Studies*, *27*, 317–330. doi:10.1007/s10899-010-9209-x

Straus, M. A. (1979). Measuring intrafamily conflict and violence: The Conflict Tactics (CT) scales. *Journal of Marriage and the Family*, *41*, 75–88. doi:10.2307/351733

Thompson, W. N., Gazel, R., & Rickman, D. (2012). Social costs of gambling: A comparative study of nutmeg and cheese state gamblers. *UNLV Gaming Research & Review Journal*, *5*(1), 1.

Toce-Gerstein, M., Gerstein, D. R., & Volberg, R. A. (2003). A hierarchy of gambling disorders in the community. *Addiction, 98*, 1661–1672. doi:10.1111/j.1360-0443.2003.00545.x

Welte, J. W., Barnes, G. M., Tidwell, M. C., & Hoffman, J. H. (2008). The prevalence of problem gambling among U.S. adolescents and young adults: Results from a national survey. *Journal of Gambling Studies*, *24*, 119–133. doi:10.1007/s10899-007-9086-0

Wildeman, C., Emanuel, N., Leventhal, J. M., Putnam-Hornstein, E., Waldfogel, J., & Lee, H. (2014). The prevalence of confirmed maltreatment among us children, 2004 to 2011. *JAMA Pediatrics*, *168*, 706–713. doi:10.1001/jamapediatrics.2014.410

Wyatt, G. E. (1985). The sexual abuse of Afro-American and White-American women in childhood. *Child Abuse and Neglect, 9*, 507–519. doi:http://dx.doi.org/10.1016/0145-2134(85)90060-2

The Effects of Childhood Sexual Abuse and Other Trauma on Drug Court Participants

MOLLY R. WOLF, PhD, LMSW
Adjunct Assistant Professor, Social Work Department, Edinboro University of Pennsylvania, Edinboro, Pennsylvania, USA

THOMAS H. NOCHAJSKI, PhD
Research Professor, School of Social Work, University at Buffalo, The State University of New York, Buffalo, New York, USA

HON. MARK G. FARRELL, JD
Retired Senior Justice, Town of Amherst, Amherst Therapeutic Drug Court, Amherst, New York, USA

Within the context of a larger study of drug court participants, this study examined the impact of traumatic experiences on psychiatric distress and on court outcomes. In the analyses, the participants (n = 229) were separated into 3 groups: childhood sexual abuse (CSA; n = 18), other trauma (n = 134), and no trauma (n = 77). The CSA group had higher mean scores on depression, anxiety, panic disorder, social phobia, somatization, and posttraumatic stress disorder than the other trauma group. Path analyses suggest that a history of trauma is a positive predictor of psychiatric distress and negative court events (positive urine screens, sanctions, etc.), with indirect effects on substance abuse severity, and failure in the drug court. These results suggest a need for the initial assessment procedure in drug courts to include a screening for trauma history, including CSA. They also suggest a need for trauma-informed care within drug courts.

Child sexual abuse (CSA) is a widespread problem that affects one in every four girls (Dube et al., 2005). A recent meta-analysis of prevalence rates of CSA suggests that almost 8% of males and almost 20% of females have been the victims of CSA (Pereda, Guilera, Forns, & Gomez-Benito, 2009). In 2000, there were approximately 88,000 substantiated cases of CSA, and these constituted about 10% of all officially reported child abuse cases (Putnam, 2003). The children in these cases, who were 4 years of age or older at the time of reporting thc abuse in 2000, would all be approaching the age of majority in 2014. These reported cases represent only a portion of the actual cases of CSA that have occurred, as only a fraction of all cases of CSA are reported. Research suggests that only about half of all victims disclose the abuse to anyone (Putnam, 2003).

CHILD SEXUAL ABUSE, CHILD ABUSE, AND SUBSTANCE USE AND ABUSE

In general, there is a link between surviving child abuse as a child and growing up to become addicted to substances (Conroy, Degenhardt, Mattick, & Nelson, 2009; Felitti, 2004). In fact, evidence from the Adverse Childhood Experiences study suggests that "the compulsive use of nicotine, alcohol, and injected street drugs increases proportionally in a strong, graded, dose-response manner that closely parallels the intensity of adverse life experiences during childhood" (Felitti, 2004, p. 3). The link between CSA history and adolescent and adult substance use and misuse is well established, whether it be illegal narcotics or alcohol (Branstetter, Bower, Kamien, & Amass, 2008; Brems, Johnson, Neal, & Freemon, 2005; Ouimette, Kimerling, Shaw, & Moos, 2000). Research suggests that a history of CSA can be associated with earlier age of onset for drug abuse (Ompad et al., 2005), increased risk for alcohol dependence (Clay, Olsheski, & Clay, 2000; Sartor et al., 2007), and a lesser response to treatment (Boles, Joshi, Grella, & Wellisch, 2005; Sacks, McKendrick, & Banks, 2008).

Gender appears to play a significant role in the relationship between CSA and substance abuse (Conroy et al., 2009; Hyman et al., 2008; Klanecky, Harrington, & McChargue, 2008; Nehls & Sallmann, 2005). Conroy et al. (2009) found that whereas males with opioid dependence in their study had suffered from physical abuse, emotional abuse, or both in childhood, the females who were opioid dependent were more likely to have suffered CSA. Females with a history of CSA can present with more psychiatric issues than those without a history of abuse, which can make treatment for both the CSA as well as the substance abuse more difficult than if the client presented with either issue alone (Branstetter et al., 2008). The combination of CSA and substance abuse can be particularly problematic in females, as research suggests that such females can experience slower recovery times or even less recovery overall than females without a history of abuse (Branstetter et al., 2008). Siegel and Williams (2003) used a prospective methodology to study the trajectory for female survivors of CSA and crimes committed in adulthood. These women had all visited the hospital in childhood as a result of CSA, and these researchers discovered that they were more likely to be arrested in adulthood for drug crimes than their matched nonabused counterparts (in the control group).

DRUG COURTS

The establishment of a court specifically for crimes relating to substance use and abuse was introduced into the United States in 1989 (Cooper, 2003). There are now more than 2,600 "drug courts" in the United States and there are many specialties within the prototype of drug courts, such as drug courts for veterans, drug courts for juveniles, tribal drug courts, and DUI courts (National Institute of Justice, 2012). It is the task of drug courts to function under the paradigm of rehabilitation, instead of using the courts as a punitive tool of justice (Turner et al., 2002). Drug courts operate with the understanding that offenders can come to the court system with a variety of psychological issues besides the presenting problem of substance use or misuse (Turner et al., 2002). Under this paradigm, the drug courts do not use incarceration as a first option, and instead use substance abuse treatment programs as a tool for therapeutic jurisprudence (Belenko, 2001). Whereas drug courts generally have a 50% graduation rate (Belenko, 2001), parole and probation generally show a 30% rate of retention (Marlowe, 2003). Furthermore, a recent meta-analysis suggests that drug courts are effective at reducing reoffenses (Mitchell, Wilson, Eggers, & MacKenzie, 2014).

TRAUMATIC STRESS AND TREATMENT FOR SUBSTANCE ABUSE IN DRUG COURTS

The majority of females who are incarcerated are there for drug-related offenses (Bureau of Justice Statistics, 2005), and the number of arrests for drug-related offenses has almost doubled in the last 20 years (Bureau of Justice Statistics, 2007). A significant portion of drug court participants tend to have a history of trauma exposure, including child abuse, and this is especially so for female participants (Kang, Magura, Laudet, & Whitney, 1999; Sartor et al., 2012; Schumacher, Coffey, & Stasiewicz, 2006). For those who have experienced trauma, posttraumatic stress symptoms become another challenge. Some survivors cope by using legal and illegal substances as an emotional anesthetic for their trauma symptoms (Brady, Back, & Coffey, 2004). The link between posttraumatic symptoms and abuse of such substances has been well-established (Back et al., 2000; Dvorak, Arens, Kuvaas, Williams, & Kilwein, 2013; Holbrook, Galarneau, Dye, Quinn, & Dougherty, 2010; Wiechelt, Miller, Smyth, & Maguin, 2011), and living with the aftereffects of a traumatic experience can have a severe effect on treatment outcomes for drug court participants (Mills, Teesson, Ross, & Darke, 2007). Dissociation is a common coping mechanism for trauma survivors, and there is a link between trauma history and dissociation through substance abuse for females (Klanecky et al., 2008; Najavits & Walsh, 2012; Nehls & Sallmann, 2005). However, Sartor et al. (2012) found that although the majority of females in drug courts had suffered previous trauma, the presence of posttraumatic stress disorder (PTSD) was not significantly associated with outcomes such as prostitution or homelessness. Instead, that study found that it was the exposure to trauma itself that was significantly associated with such outcomes.

Although it is common for women with substance abuse issues or mental health problems to have a history of trauma (Fallot & Harris, 2005; McHugo et al., 2005; Savage, Quiros, Dodd, & Bonavota, 2007), substance abuse issues are not being addressed in settings that treat sexual abuse (Zweig, Schlichter, & Burt, 2002) even though severity of PTSD symptoms (specifically the symptom of reexperiencing) is a significant predictor of relapse for substance abuse (Brown, 2000). However, when treating these women, it has been just as common to concentrate only on the substance abuse or the mental health problems, without giving much credence to the cause of these issues (i.e., the trauma; Blakely & Bowers, 2014). It has long been thought that if the addiction is treated simultaneously with the trauma history, the two issues will compete with each other and the addiction will lose, causing the client to abuse substances again (Blakely & Bowers, 2014). However, in a study on a trauma-focused intervention, the Trauma Recovery and Empowerment Model (TREM) was found to have no differential effect on relapse prevention, but had a beneficial impact on trauma symptoms (Toussaint, VanDeMark, Bornemann, & Graeber, 2007). Furthermore, studies suggest that a different trauma-focused intervention, Seeking Safety, is beneficial for trauma survivors who have substance abuse issues (Najavits, Gallop, & Weiss, 2006; Najavits, Schmitz, Gotthardt, & Weiss, 2005). Other studies have echoed these findings, which would suggest that it is actually better for the client to have integrated trauma and addiction services, but only if using an evidence-based approach (McHugo et al., 2005; Savage et al., 2007; Toussaint et al., 2007). These results suggest that it would be beneficial to conceptualize treatment for a trauma survivor with chemical addiction as not only treatment for the addiction, but also the issues that might have led to the addiction.

In their review of treatment options for female offenders with substance abuse issues, Adams, Leukefeld, and Peden (2008) recommended empowerment, social support networks, and collaboration as key aspects in the care and treatment for this population. These are also key aspects of trauma-informed care (Fallot & Harris, 2006). The idea behind trauma-informed care in an environment such as a drug court is that it is not necessarily plausible to know which defendants are trauma survivors and which are not, but it is best to assume that everyone in the court has been exposed to trauma, and to use a trauma-informed approach with all involved (Elliott, Bjelajac, Fallot, Markoff, & Reed, 2005). Trauma-informed care can be used in combination with trauma-specific care or on its own (Elliott et al., 2005), and has been shown to be effective in treatment for substance abuse (Amaro et al., 2004).

AIM OF THE THIS STUDY

This study examined the impact of traumatic experiences on drug court participants. It made a specific distinction between CSA and other traumatic experiences to determine if the individuals who experienced CSA had more negative outcomes than those who experienced other types of trauma, and if those with other trauma experiences had more negative outcomes than those who did not experience any traumatic event. The hypothesis of this research was that drug court participants with a history of CSA would be more likely to deal with a larger number of psychosocial problems than their peers who have suffered from other types of trauma, or when compared to nontrauma survivors. A secondary aim of the study was to test whether the CSA would directly or indirectly influence failure in the drug court when controlling for gender, alcohol problem severity, drug problem severity, psychological distress, and negative drug court events (positive urine screens, being sanctioned, or out on warrant).

METHODS

Participants

Potential participants for this study were individuals referred to the drug court in western New York. Eligible participants were over 18, did not have any past violent offenses, and did not have serious mental illness at the time of intake. Of the 396 individuals initially referred to the drug court, 230 were interviewed (58%) for this study. One participant's information was not used in the final analyses due to missing data, so the final number of participants was 229. Using information from the drug court screen, comparison between the individuals who entered the study and those who did not showed no differences for gender, race, prior criminal history, history of drug use other than opiates, suicide attempts, disability, number of sanctions, or failure in the drug court. However, the group of individuals who did not enter the study were older (35 vs. 31; $p = .003$); more likely to have been out on warrant (63.5% vs. 47.0%; $p = .001$); more likely to have a history of opiate problems (33% vs. 21%; $p = .008$); had more alcohol problems (4.92 vs. 3.89; $p = .02$); and had more drug problems (6.29 vs. 4.02; $p < .001$). Individuals who entered the study were more likely to have a current charge of a DWI (46% vs. 22%; $p < .001$); have a positive toxicology report (48% vs. 24%; $p < .001$); and to have mental health problems (19% vs. 10%; $p = .024$). Thus the two groups were different on some important variables, indicating a need for caution when interpreting the findings.

Measures

This study used the Beck Anxiety Inventory (BAI; Beck, Epstein, Brown, & Steer, 1988), the Beck Depression Inventory–II (BDI; Beck, Steer, & Brown, 1996), drug and alcohol screening instruments, and several measures to identify mental health status of the participants.

The BAI is a 21-item scale that measures severity of anxiety. It uses a Likert-based scale with responses ranging from not at all to severely. For this study, the alpha coefficient was .935. In addition to the total score, this study also considered the recommended cutpoints to identify individuals who would be considered moderate or severely anxious (scores 16 and above). The BDI is a 21-item scale that measures the symptoms of depression. The BDI provides four response options for each question with the options representing low, mild, moderate, and severe risk for depression. The total score can then be broken down into risk level categories. For the purposes of this study, the total score was dichotomized into severe and extreme depression versus all other categories. Additionally, the total score was considered. The alpha coefficient for the scale was .944.

For substance use, the drug court screen was a 32-question measure: 16 questions focusing on alcohol-related problems, used in this study to measure alcohol problem severity ($\alpha = .878$), and 16 focusing on problems with drugs other than alcohol used as the measure of drug problem severity ($\alpha = .924$). In addition, the drug court screen was used to identify the number of substances used, and whether the individual had a history of problems. Specific substances considered were alcohol, cannabis, cocaine or crack, and heroin or opiates. The age of first problem use was also asked for each substance identified. For the current study the youngest age was used to reflect age at first use.

Mental health status was assessed using a number of different measures. The Psychiatric Diagnostic Screening Questionnaire (PDSQ; Zimmerman & Mattia, 1999) is a 125-item instrument that assesses a range of Axis I disorders from the *Diagnostic and Statistical Manual of Mental Disorders* (4th ed. [*DSM–IV*]; American Psychiatric Association, 2000). This study used the major depression ($\alpha = .894$), PTSD ($\alpha = .953$), bulimia ($\alpha = .909$), obsessive–compulsive ($\alpha = .856$), panic disorder ($\alpha = .868$), social phobia (α = .894), generalized anxiety (α = .928), agoraphobia (α = .890), and somatization subscales (α = .606), as well as total for the aforementioned subscales, excluding PTSD (α = .965). In addition to the total scores for the respective subscales, the instrument also allows for identification of high risk for diagnosis in the respective areas using cutpoints determined with previous nonclinical samples. These were used in this study along with the total subscale scores to gain a better understanding of how trauma influences psychological distress.

For purposes of the assessment of the indirect effects of trauma exposure and psychological distress on failure in the drug court, the scores from the eight subscales mentioned for the PDSQ previously, excluding PTSD, were summed and then the z score was calculated. The z scores were also calculated for the BDI and BAI. All z scores were then summed to use as the overall measure of psychological distress.

The Modified PTSD Symptom Scale–Self Report (MPSS; Falsetti, Resnick, Resick, & Kilpatrick, 1993) was used to provide an assessment of PTSD symptoms for the offenders. The instrument is a 17 item self-report measure that assesses the *DSM–IV* symptoms of PTSD. The individuals are asked to provide frequency and intensity of the symptoms on Likert scales ranging from 0 (*not at all*) to 3 (*5 or more times per week*) for the frequency and 0 (*not at all distressing*) to 4 (*extremely distressing*) for severity. There are three subscales in the instrument: reexperiencing, arousal, and avoidance. The scores were constructed by summing the frequency and intensity items. The alpha coefficient for the total scale frequency score was .978. Subscale scores for the reexperiencing (criterion B), avoidance and numbing (criterion C), and hyperarousal (criterion D) were also computed. Alpha coefficients were .921, .958, and .955 for the reexeperiencing, avoidance numbing, and hyperarousal criteria, respectively.

Exposure to traumatic events was determined using the drug court screening information and the MPSS, as well as the PDSQ. In the study sample, 77 individuals did not indicate trauma experiences of any kind, 134 indicated they had experienced some type of traumatic event that did not involve CSA, and 18 indicated some type of CSA.

Suicidal ideation was constructed from the questions in the drug screen, as well as the items in the PDSQ and BDI that refer to thoughts of suicide. A positive response on any item was considered a yes. The demographics included age, gender, race or ethnicity, marital status, education level, and employment status. In addition, prior criminal history (yes or no) and the current charge (theft, possession, DWI) were also considered.

Data Analysis

Trauma exposure was measured by splitting the sample into three groups: no trauma, other trauma (except CSA), and CSA. Bivariate associations between trauma exposure and all other variables were performed using crosstabs with chi-square and logistic regression for dichotomous variables, and one-way analyses of variance for continuous variables. Levene's test for homogeneity of variance was used to determine if group variances were significantly different from one another. If they were, then the Welch test was used to determine significance. Bonferroni adjustments were made considering the number of tests performed within each category. Post-hoc analyses were considered for all significant associations to determine group differences. Bonferroni adjustments were also used for this purpose.

Subsequent to the bivariate associations, we tested a model of how CSA influenced drug court outcomes. Path analysis was performed using *Mplus* version 7.1. The model tested is shown in Figure 1. To assess model fit, the following goodness-of-fit measures were used: the likelihood ratio chi-square statistic ($p > .05$), the comparative fit index (CFI > .95), the Tucker–Lewis index (TLI > .95), the root mean square error of approximation (RMSEA < .06), and the weighted root mean square residual (WRMR < .8). To reduce bias, bias-corrected bootstrapping was used to calculate the confidence intervals (CIs) for the parameters.

In terms of power, we recognize that the CSA group was relatively small and so power would be an issue for any group comparisons. For the bivariate comparisons there was an average effect size of around .3 for overall tests, suggesting that a small to moderate effect size was common. Given the consistency in our results, we feel that the power was sufficient for detecting the group differences. For the path analysis, we also recognize that the CSA group had only 18 individuals, meaning that our power would be reduced for the overall path model. However, in using the bias-corrected bootstrapping method to build standard errors to test the parameters, we feel that the results presented show there was sufficient power to establish relatively stable path coefficients.

RESULTS

Bivariate comparisons across demographic characteristics showed significant differences only for gender (see Table 1). The no trauma and other trauma groups showed similar percentages for women; in contrast, individuals in the CSA group were more than nine times more likely than the no trauma group to be female.

There was a clear linear trend concerning prior arrests (see Table 2). Whereas 63.6% of nontraumatized participants had prior arrest records, 76.9% of other trauma survivors and 94.4% of CSA survivors had prior arrest records. At the same time, the results of this study suggest an opposite trend for current DWI: Whereas almost half of the participants without a trauma

TABLE 1 Bivariate Comparisons Between Trauma Exposure and Demographic Characteristics

	No trauma ($n = 77$) n (%)	Other trauma ($n = 134$) n (%)	CSA ($n = 18$) n (%)	Significance
Gender (Female)*	17 (22.1)[a]	34 (25.4)[a]	13 (72.2)[b]	$\chi^2(2, N = 229) = 19.28, p < .001$
Age				*ns*
M	31.77	31.50	35.44	
SD	11.34	10.68	10.42	
Race (White)	63 (81.8)	100 (74.6)	10 (55.6)	$\chi^2(2, N = 229) = 5.60, p = .061$
Education				
<High school	7 (9.1)	15 (11.2)	3 (16.7)	*ns*
>High school	41 (53.2)	59 (44.0)	10 (55.6)	*ns*
Marital status				
Divorced/separated/widowed	8 (10.5)	22 (16.4)	5 (27.8)	*ns*
Never married	49 (64.5)	91 (67.9)	10 (55.6)	*ns*
Unemployed	29 (39.2)	59 (45.7)	10 (58.8)	*ns*

Note: Different superscripts indicate significant differences between groups. CSA = childhood sexual abuse.
*Indicates significant at $p < .05$ level after Bonferroni adjustment.

TABLE 2 Bivariate Comparisons Between Trauma Exposure and Criminal History and Current Charges

	No trauma ($n = 77$) n (%)	Other trauma ($n = 135$) n (%)	CSA ($n = 18$) n (%)	Significance
Criminal history (Yes)*	49 (63.6)[a]	103 (76.9)[a]	17 (94.4)[b]	$\chi^2(2, N = 229) = 8.73, p = .013$
Current charge				
Theft related	9 (11.7)[a]	38 (28.4)[b]	5 (27.8)[ab]	$\chi^2(2, N = 229) = 8.029, p = .018$
Possession	24 (31.2)	40 (29.9)	9 (50.0)	*ns*
DWI*	44 (57.1)[a]	59 (44.0)[a]	2 (11.1)[b]	$\chi^2(2, N = 229) = 12.88, p = .002$

Note: Different superscripts indicate significant differences between groups. CSA = childhood sexual abuse; DWI = driving while intoxicated.
*Indicates significant at $p < .05$ level after Bonferroni adjustment.

history and with other trauma histories (57.1% and 44.0%, respectively) had current DWIs, only 11.1% of the CSA survivors had current DWIs.

Table 3 shows the substance use measures. It was clear that alcohol was more preferred by the no trauma and other trauma groups, whereas other drugs, such as marijuana, cocaine or crack, and opiates or heroin, were more preferred by the CSA group than the other two groups. It is also clear that the number of alcohol-related problems did not differ for the three

TABLE 3 Bivariate Comparisons Between Trauma Exposure and Court Record Substance Use Measures

Substances used	No trauma ($n = 75$) n (%)	Other trauma ($n = 134$) n (%)	CSA ($n = 18$) n (%)	Significance
Alcohol	73 (97.3)[a]	128 (95.5)[a]	14 (77.8)[b]	χ^2 (2, $N = 227$) = 11.51, $p = .003$
Marijuana	50 (66.7)	104 (77.6)	16 (88.9)	χ^2(2, $N = 227$) = 5.10, $p = .078$
Cocaine and/or crack	30 (40.0)[a]	69 (51.5)[ab]	13 (72.2)[b]	χ^2(2, $N = 227$) = 6.64, $p = .036$
Heroin/opiates	10 (13.3)	32 (23.9)	6 (33.3)	χ^2(2, $N = 227$) = 4.95, $p = .084$
No. problem substances				$F(2, 224) = 2.95$, $p = .054$, $\eta^2 = .026$
M	2.49	3.03	3.06	
SD	1.37	1.73	1.11	
No. alcohol problems				*ns*
M	3.19	3.39	3.06	
SD	2.84	3.51	3.72	
No. drug problems				$F(2, 48) = 6.40$, $p = .003$, $\eta^2 = .048$
M	2.71	4.69	5.44	
SD	3.88[a]	4.78[b]	4.37[b]	
Age of first use				$F(2, 224) = 2.79$, $p = .063$, $\eta^2 = .024$
M	16.56	15.54	15.11	
SD	3.94	2.79	3.66	

Note: Different superscripts indicate significant differences between groups. CSA = childhood sexual abuse.
*Indicates significant at $p < .05$ level after Bonferroni adjustment.

groups, whereas the drug problems were greater for the other trauma and CSA groups than the no trauma group.

As shown in Table 4, there is a clear linear trend for depression and anxiety scores, with CSA survivors experiencing these issues significantly more than the other trauma group and the nontrauma participants. The results also show the survivors of CSA scoring higher in social phobia, panic disorder, and bulimia than the no trauma or other trauma groups. In addition, the CSA group was significantly higher than the no trauma and other trauma groups on the total scores for the BDI and BAI.

Results considering the cutoffs for high risk of having one of the mental health disorders assessed by the PDSQ showed that the two trauma-exposed groups were more likely than the no trauma group to be at risk (Table 5). The findings for the BDI and BAI, however, show a linear trend, with the CSA survivors being at greatest risk to be in the moderate or high anxiety category or the severe or extreme depression category compared with the other trauma group, who was more likely to be identified as high risk than the no trauma group.

TABLE 4 Bivariate Comparisons Between Trauma Exposure and Measures of Psychological Distress

	No trauma (n = 77)		Other trauma (n = 134)		CSA (n = 18)		
	M	*SD*	*M*	*SD*	*M*	*SD*	Significance
PDSQ							
Depression*	2.34[a]	3.53	3.78[b]	4.37	6.89[c]	4.78	$F(2, 226) = 9.36, p < .001, \eta^2 = .076$
Generalized anxiety*	1.45[a]	2.51	2.63[b]	3.50	5.06[c]	3.62	$F(2, 226) = 9.84, p < .001, \eta^2 = .080$
Panic disorder*	0.32[a]	1.16	0.78[a]	1.85	1.94[b]	2.92	$F(2, 226) = 6.34, p = .002, \eta^2 = .053$
Agoraphobia	0.38	1.17	0.72	1.93	1.22	2.42	*ns*
Social phobia*	0.66[a]	2.02	1.42[a]	2.81	3.67[b]	4.31	$F(2, 226) = 8.96, p < .001, \eta^2 = .074$
OCD	0.21	0.70	0.60	1.53	0.50	0.86	$F(2, 226) = 2.34, p = .099, \eta^2 = .020$
Somatization	0.30[a]	0.69	0.64[b]	1.02	0.94[b]	1.11	$F(2, 226) = 5.07, p = .007, \eta^2 = .043$
Bulimia*	0.51[a]	1.48	0.51[a]	1.61	2.78[b]	3.37	$F(2, 226) = 13.67, p < .001, \eta^2 = .108$
Beck assessments							
BAI*	4.30[a]	5.76	8.50[b]	10.78	19.17[c]	12.55	$F(2, 226) = 18.24, p < .001, \eta^2 = .139$
BDI*	6.26[a]	8.35	10.62[b]	11.20	19.78[c]	13.88	$F(2, 226) = 12.74, p < .001, \eta^2 = .101$

Note: Different superscripts indicate significant differences between groups based on Bonferroni adjusted comparisons for continuous measures. CSA = childhood sexual abuse; PDSQ = Psychiatric Diagnostic Screening Questionnaire; OCD = obsessive–compulsive disorder; BAI = Beck Anxiety Inventory; BDI = Beck Depression Inventory.

*Indicates significant at $p < .05$ level after Bonferroni adjustment ($p < .005$).

The results reflected in Tables 5 and 6 show that traumatic event experiences are highly related to psychiatric distress in drug court participants. Furthermore, when considering PTSD symptoms, the CSA group scores higher than the other trauma group on all measures used for this study (see Table 6).

Moreover, there is a clear linear trend for survivors of CSA to be more likely to experience a range of negative outcomes in the drug court, such as positive urine screens, sanctions, warrants, and failure in the drug court, than were their other trauma and nontraumatized counterparts (see Table 7). A majority of the individuals with no admitted exposure to a traumatic event had a negative event in the drug court, but the percentage increased to over 75% for the other trauma group and almost 90% for the CSA survivors. Likewise, failure rates were relatively low in this drug court, reflecting the attitude of the presiding judge to allow for second and third chances before failing them out. Nonetheless, it is clear that the trauma-exposed groups were more likely to fail than the no trauma group.

TABLE 5 Bivariate Comparisons Between Trauma Exposure and Clinical Cutoffs of Psychological Distress

	No trauma ($n = 77$)		Other trauma ($n = 134$)		CSA ($n = 18$)		
	%	n	%	n	%	n	Significance
Thoughts of suicide	9.2%	7^{a}	21.6%	29^{b}	33.3%	6^{b}	$\chi^2(2, N = 229) = 8.075, p = .018$
PDSQ							
Depression	11.7%	9^{a}	16.3%	22^{ab}	33.3%	6^{b}	$\chi^2(2, N = 229) = 5.06, p = .080$
Generalized anxiety	6.5%	5^{a}	20.1%	27^{b}	33.3%	6^{b}	$\chi^2(2, N = 229) = 10.54, p = .005$
Panic disorder	2.6%	2^{a}	8.2%	11^{ab}	22.2%	4^{b}	$\chi^2(2, N = 229) = 8.47, p = .015$
Agoraphobia	5.2%	4	12.7%	17	11.1%	2	*ns*
Social phobia*	7.8%	6^{a}	15.7%	21^{a}	44.4%	8^{b}	$\chi^2(2, N = 229) = 15.12, p = .001$
OCD	10.4%	8^{a}	20.9%	28^{ab}	33.3%	6^{b}	$\chi^2(2, N = 229) = 6.54, p = .038$
Somatization*	3.9%	3^{a}	17.9%	24^{b}	33.3%	6^{b}	$\chi^2(2, N = 229) = 13.46, p = .001$
Bulimia*	1.3%	1^{a}	3.0%	4^{a}	16.7%	3^{b}	$\chi^2(2, N = 229) = 10.47, p = .005$
Beck assessments							
BAI*	1.3%	1^{a}	11.2%	15^{b}	44.4%	8^{c}	$\chi^2(2, N = 229) = 29.12, p < .001$
BDI*	1.3%	1^{a}	8.2%	11^{b}	22.2%	4^{c}	$\chi^2(2, N = 229) = 10.57, p = .005$

Note: For anxiety the breakdown was low anxiety versus moderate or high; for depression the comparison was severe and extreme against all other categories. Different superscripts indicate significant differences between groups based on Bonferroni adjusted comparisons for continuous measures. CSA = childhood sexual abuse; PDSQ = Psychiatric Diagnostic Screening Questionnaire; OCD = obsessive–compulsive disorder; BAI = Beck Anxiety Inventory; BDI = Beck Depression Inventory.
*Indicates significant at $p < .05$ level after Bonferroni adjustment.

These results show that traumatic events can have effects on factors that are critical to success in the drug court. It is also clear that CSA survivors tend to have more negative outcomes than the no trauma and other trauma groups. The next analysis considers how the CSA event might influence the important areas for succeeding in drug courts. For the final analysis, a model was developed based on findings from the literature and these results. This model suggests that CSA impacts drug court outcomes through psychiatric distress, which then results in problem use of alcohol, drugs, or both. This problematic use of alcohol, drugs, or both then leads to negative outcomes in the drug court. This model was tested using M*plus* version 7.1, with bootstrap methods using 10,000 replications to build the standard errors and CIs for the indirect effects.

TABLE 6 Bivariate Comparisons Between Trauma Exposure and PTSD Symptoms

	Other trauma exposure ($n = 134$)	Childhood sexual abuse ($n = 18$)	Significance
Number of traumatic events	3.23 (2.18)	4.28 (2.78)	$t(150) = -1.85, p = .066, \eta^2 = .102$
PDSQ PTSD scale*	2.49 (3.79)	6.61 (5.25)	$t(19) = -3.22, p = .004, \eta^2 = .102$
PDSQ PTSD CUT	18.7% ($n = 25$)	55.6% ($n = 10$)	$\chi^2(1, N = 153) = 12.19, p < .001$
PTSD scale			
Rexperiencing*	3.00 (6.27)	9.94 (9.16)	$t(19) = -3.22, p = .004, \eta^2 = .103$
Avoidance/numbing	4.37 (9.76)	10.39 (12.40)	$t(150) = -2.38, p = .019, \eta^2 = .036$
Arousal	3.25 (7.80)	7.44 (8.50)	$t(150) = -2.12, p = .036, \eta^2 = .029$
Total*	10.62 (22.64)	27.78 (27.58)	$t(150) = -2.94, p = .004, \eta^2 = .054$

Note: PTSD = posttraumatic stress disorder; PDSQ = PDSQ = Psychiatric Diagnostic Screening Questionnaire.
*Indicates significant at $p < .05$ level after Bonferroni adjustment for number of tests in this table.

TABLE 7 Bivariate Comparisons for Trauma Exposure and Drug Court Program Measures

	No trauma ($n = 77$)		Other trauma ($n = 134$)		CSA ($n = 18$)		
	n	%	n	%	n	%	Significance
Positive urine screens*	26	33.8[a]	72	53.7[b]	12	66.7[b]	$\chi^2(2, N = 299) = 10.53, p = .005$
Sanctions*	30	39.0[a]	75	56.0[b]	14	77.8[b]	$\chi^2(2, N = 299) = 10.82, p = .004$
Bench warrants	31	40.3[a]	64	47.8[a]	13	72.2[b]	$\chi^2(2, N = 299) = 6.03, p = .049$
Any negative event	44	57.1	102	76.1	16	88.9	$\chi^2(2, N = 299) = 11.62, p = .003$
Failed drug court	11	14.3[a]	36	26.9[b]	7	38.9[b]	$\chi^2(2, N = 299) = 6.35, p = .033$

Note: Different superscripts indicate significant differences between groups based on Bonferroni adjusted comparisons for continuous measures. CSA = childhood sexual abuse.
*Indicates significant at $p < .05$ level after Bonferroni adjustment.

Table 8 shows the correlations between the measures used in the path analysis. Gender was included and showed significant associations with CSA and psychological distress. Psychological distress shows associations with alcohol problems, drug problems, negative drug court events, and failure. Drug problems were associated with negative drug court events and failure

TABLE 8 Correlations for Measures Used in Path Analyses for Failure in Drug Court

	2	3	4	5	6	7
1. Gender	.288***	.369***	−.032	.052	.101	.067
2. Childhood sexual abuse	—	.303***	−.021	.087	.117	.105
3. Psychological disturbance		—	.298***	.331***	.150*	.190**
4. Alcohol problems			—	.210**	−.017	−.034
5. Drug problems				—	.274***	.341***
6. Any negative event					—	.335***
7. Failed						—

Note: $N = 229$.
*$p < .05$. **$p < .01$. ***$p < .001$.

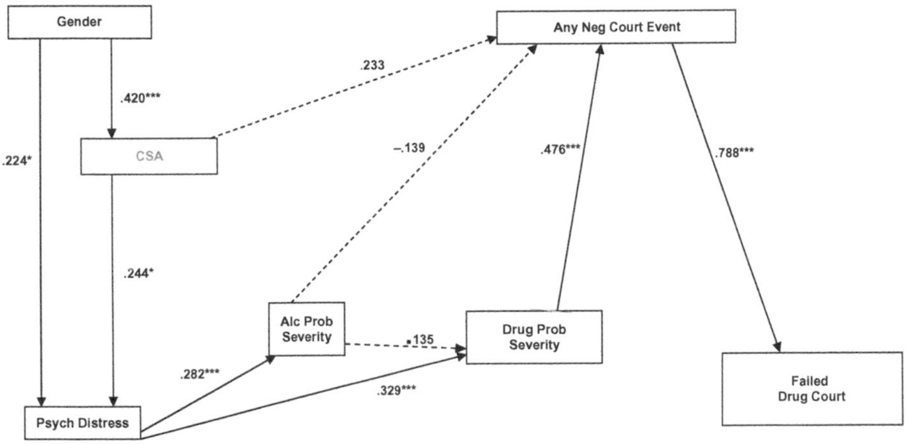

FIGURE 1 Model for path analysis. *Note:* CSA = childhood sexual abuse.

in the drug court, with, as might be expected, negative drug court events being associated with failure in the drug court.

The model fit was good for the analysis, with the chi-square being non-significant ($p = .4636$), the CFI being 1, the TLI being 1, RMSEA being .000, and the WRMR being .527. Figure 1 shows the final model with standardized path coefficients. Significant paths are noted. When using the bias-corrected bootstrap standard errors, the two paths involving alcohol predictions (alcohol to negative drug court events and alcohol to drug problems) did not fall within the 95% or 90% CI and the CSA to negative outcomes parameter estimate fell within the 90% CI.

Indirect paths were assessed using the bias-corrected standard errors to determine CIs for the coefficients. Of specific interest were indirect effects from CSA to failure in the drug court, negative events in the drug court, drug problems, and alcohol problems. The CI for the parameter estimate (.030) for the indirect path from CSA to psychological distress to drug problems to negative court events (e.g., positive urine screens) to failure in the drug court fell within the 90% CI [.001, .059]. The parameter (.184) for the indirect path from CSA to negative court events to failure in the drug court also fell in the 90% CI [.011, .357]. Thus, there was marginal support for an indirect effect of CSA on failure in the drug court.

When considering the indirect pathway for psychological distress, the parameter (.123) for the psychological distress to drug problems to negative court events to failure in the drug court fell within the 95% CI [.014, .233]. Finally, the parameter (.375) for the indirect path from drug problems to negative court events to failure in the drug court fell within the 99% CI [.101, 648]. None of the indirect paths for alcohol problems showed indications of possible relationships, suggesting that the failure in drug courts is not a function of the alcohol problems; rather it is more a function of the drug problems that showed a strong association with CSA.

DISCUSSION

The hypothesis in this research study was that participants with a history of CSA would fare worse than participants with other trauma history or without any trauma history. The results of this study supported this hypothesis. There was a clear linear trend for negative outcomes from participants without a trauma history, to participants with a trauma history, to participants with a CSA history. These findings suggest that participants with a trauma history, and specifically those with a history of surviving CSA, have more negative outcomes in and out of drug court than participants without any trauma history at all. The linear trend shows that although participants with a trauma history are more likely to fail drug court, have a positive urine screen, sanctions, warrants, depression, bulimia, obsessive–compulsive disorder, agoraphobia, social phobia, generalized anxiety, and elevated mental health scores, participants who are survivors of CSA are even more likely to experience these negative outcomes.

The results of this study suggest that any traumatic experience puts a drug court participant at increased risk for failure and other consequences, and a history of CSA seems to magnify that risk. These risk factors indicate a need for different forms of interventions for trauma and CSA survivors than those that can be used for standard drug court participants. The results from the path analysis indicate that CSA and psychological distress have indirect effects on failure in drug courts, with indirect effects on alcohol and drug problems through psychological distress. Given the temporal ordering of the CSA and substance use this is a logical outcome.

The CSA survivors in this study were significantly more likely to experience panic disorder, anxiety, agoraphobia, and social phobia. Simply put, these survivors were more panicked and afraid than their other trauma counterparts in drug courts, even those who had experienced traumas as severe as witnessing murder or being raped (in adulthood). When compared to other trauma survivors, CSA survivors scored higher on three particular areas of the PTSD scale: reexperiencing, avoidance/numbing, and arousal. These results suggest that there is something uniquely dangerous about experiencing incest, CSA, or both (as compared to other traumas) that, if untreated, have lifelong negative implications. Being a powerless child and experiencing the abuse of one's own body has left these survivors with a more difficult path in terms of recovery from substance abuse.

It is important to note that the participants in the CSA group experienced many of the other traumas experienced by the other trauma group. This would mean that unfortunately the CSA survivors not only experienced CSA, but also a range of traumas adding to a long line of betrayals against them (Gold, 2000; 2002). In fact this was shown in Table 6, but importantly, the other trauma group also showed more than one traumatic experience. Thus, the small CSA group in this study is probably representative of most CSA survivors. In this vein, the CSA could be conceptualized as either one of many terrible things that happened to the participant, or in the context of the results of this study, it could be thought of as the critical factor that led to worse outcomes than for non-CSA survivors.

Study Limitations

A major limitation of this study is the small number of participants (n = 18) with a CSA history. This number is too small to be generalizable to the general population of drug court participants with a CSA history. However, it is important to note that there is a good possibility that there were actually more CSA survivors in this study than were actually identified, because the instrument used did not ask specifically about instances of sexual abuse. Instead, the original focus of the study was the effects of trauma on drug court participants. Only those participants who took the time to write down "sexual abuse" as part of their answer to a question regarding all traumas were included in this study. Thus, another method of assessing specifically for CSA might have yielded different results. Also, although the number was small, the consistency of higher levels of pathological problems suggest that CSA is a problem worthy of further investigation and an important issue for the courts to consider.

Another potential limitation was the inability to truly assess gender differences within the context of the trauma groups. We recognize that gender is associated with CSA but our data set had too few males and too few females in other groups to perform analyses that would provide insights for how gender might have influenced the outcomes. However, we did use gender as a control variable in the path analyses and we also looked at direct associations of gender with a variety of measures. We found no association of gender with criminal history, age of first use, preferred substance, number of alcohol or drug problems, positive urine screens, sanctions, warrants, any negative outcome, or failure in the drug court. Furthermore, as shown in Table 4, there were significant differences between the no trauma and other trauma groups for depression, anxiety, and somatization, and given that the distribution of females in these two groups was equivalent, we felt that trauma was the more critical variable.

IMPLICATIONS FOR PRACTICE AND FURTHER RESEARCH

One interpretation of this research might be that substance abuse serves as a vehicle that allows survivors of CSA to dissociate and escape from the emotional pain that can accompany the survival of abuse. In other words, perhaps these substances are being used in a medicinal way to soothe away the emotional pains of childhood trauma. In viewing this issue through a strengths-based perspective, these survivors have found a coping mechanism that has facilitated an escape from unthinkable emotional pain. As CSA is an experience whereby the victim generally feels powerless, substance abuse might represent an attempt to take back the power and "control" their emotions. Indeed, Najavits and Walsh (2012) found that there was a tendency among highly dissociative women with substance abuse issues to assume that substances are beneficial in handling their psychiatric symptoms. Unfortunately, the use of substances can become a dangerous vehicle for this type of emotion control. Clinical social workers can be particularly helpful with survivors of CSA who have substance abuse issues by teaching them new and safe coping skills to replace the maladaptive coping skill of using substances to dissociate from overwhelming negative emotion. As such, this research adds to the growing body of literature that suggests a need for "trauma-focused" treatment. The results of a recent family drug court study suggest that trauma-specific care is effective in not only reducing the trauma symptoms, but also at reducing substance abuse (Powell, Stevens, Lo Dolce, Sinclair, & Swenson-Smith, 2012). If nothing else, it certainly shows a clear need for trauma-informed care when dealing with drug court participants.

A history of child abuse (including CSA) can have a severe effect on treatment outcomes for drug court participants (Kang et al., 1999). Some researchers have surmised that such treatment outcomes might be due to the fact that survivors of CSA tend to have trust issues, and thus have difficulty forming the therapeutic alliance that is necessary for effective treatment (Rosen, Ouimette, Sheikh, Gregg, & Moos, 2002). Perhaps these types of trust issues provide an explanation for the fact that social phobia was a major issue for CSA survivors in this study, in that if people have a hard time trusting others, they would also be wary of others. This can make treatment difficult, especially in terms of the usual protocol of group therapy for people with substance abuse issues. If a CSA survivor is experiencing severe panic and social phobia, it would be difficult to convince this person that group therapy (for either substance abuse, sexual abuse, or both) would be beneficial. As such, treating CSA survivors with substance abuse issues can be a challenging task, especially in a drug court situation with limited resources. However, just because a task is challenging does not mean it is not worthy, and it certainly does not mean that it is impossible. This is an opportunity for social workers to help clients work through the challenges of social phobias to help survivors feel empowered.

Perhaps early intervention for the CSA survivor would be beneficial so that traumagenic issues are worked on before a substance abuse problem even begins. Of course, this can be difficult as CSA generally happens in an environment with no witnesses, so helping professionals are reliant on the survivor himself or herself coming forward and asking for help. However, when child or adolescent survivors do present for treatment, a qualified professional who is abreast of the latest therapeutic interventions for CSA survivors might be able to help them understand the deleterious effects that alcohol and drugs might have on them later in life.

Future research might examine the relative usefulness of early intervention for trauma survivors in drug courts, particularly in terms of not only court outcomes, but also mental health outcomes. Future research should also examine the role of early intervention in trauma survivors to ascertain whether such intervention can prevent substance abuse altogether. Overall, this study suggests that there is a clear need for comprehensive assessment and treatment for drug court participants, especially for those who have experienced trauma, CSA, or both. Because trauma survivors present with many issues in addition to the presenting problem of substance abuse, there is a need for trained mental health and drug court professionals to understand the role that trauma plays in the lives of substance-abusing individuals.

FUNDING

This study received funding from the Robert Wood Johnson Foundation's Substance Abuse Policy Research Program.

REFERENCES

Adams, S., Leukefeld, C. G., & Peden, A. R. (2008). Substance abuse treatment for women offenders: A research review. *Journal of Addictions Nursing*, *19*, 61–75.

Amaro, H., McGraw, S., Larson, M. J., Lopez, L., Nieves, R., & Marshall, B. (2004). Boston Consortium of Services for Families in Recovery: A trauma-informed intervention model for women's alcohol and drug addiction treatment. *Alcoholism Treatment Quarterly*, *22*(3), 95–119.

American Psychiatric Association. (2000). *Diagnostic and statistical manual of mental disorders* (4th ed.). Washington, DC: Author.

Back, M. A., Dansky, B. S., Coffey, S. F., Saladin, M. E., Sonne, S., & Brady, K. T. (2000). Cocaine dependence with and without post-traumatic stress disorder: A comparison of substance use, trauma history, and psychiatric comorbidity. *The American Journal on Addictions*, *9*(1), 51–62.

Beck, A. T., Epstein, N., Brown, G., & Steer, R. A. (1988). An inventory for measuring clinical anxiety: Psychometric properties. *Journal of Consulting and Clinical Psychology*, *56*(6), 893–897.

Beck, A. T., Steer, R. A., & Brown, G. K. (1996). *BDI-II manual*. San Antonio, TX: Psychological Corporation.

Belenko, S. (2001). *Research on drug courts: A critical review: 2001 update*. New York, NY: National Center on Addiction and Substance Abuse at Columbia University. Retrieved from http://www.drugpolicy.org/docUploads/2001drugcourts.pdf

Blakely, J. M., & Bowers, P. H. (2014). Barriers to integrated treatment of substance abuse and trauma among women. *Journal of Social Work Practice in the Addictions*, *14*, 250–272. doi:10.1080/1533256X.2014.933731

Boles, S. M., Joshi, V., Grella, C., & Wellisch, J. (2005). Childhood sexual abuse patterns, psychosocial correlates, and treatment outcomes among adults in drug abuse treatment. *Journal of Child Sexual Abuse*, *14*, 39–55.

Brady, K. T., Back, S. E., & Coffey, S. F. (2004). Substance abuse and post-traumatic stress disorder. *Current Directions in Psychological Science*, *13*, 206–209.

Branstetter, S. A., Bower, E. H., Kamien, J., & Amass, L. (2008). A history of sexual, emotional, or physical abuse predicts adjustment during opioid maintenance treatment. *Journal of Substance Abuse Treatment*, *34*, 208–214.

Brems, C., Johnson, M. E., Neal, D., & Freemon, M. (2005). Childhood abuse history and substance use among men and women receiving detoxification services. *The American Journal of Drug and Alcohol Abuse*, *30*, 799–821.

Brown, P. J. (2000). Outcome in female patients with both substance use and post-traumatic stress disorders. *Alcoholism Treatment Quarterly*, *18*, 127–135.

Bureau of Justice Statistics. (2005). *Prison statistics: Summary findings on December 31, 2005*. Washington, DC: U.S. Department of Justice. Retrieved from http://www.bjs.gov/content/dcf/enforce.cfm

Bureau of Justice Statistics. (2007). *Drug and crime facts*. Washington, DC: U.S. Department of Justice. Retrieved from http://www.bjs.gov/content/dcf/enforce.cfm

Clay, K. M., Olsheski, J. A., & Clay, S. W. (2000). Alcohol use disorders in female survivors of childhood sexual abuse. *Alcoholism Treatment Quarterly*, *18*(4), 19–29.

Conroy, E., Degenhardt, L., Mattick, R. P., & Nelson, E. C. (2009). Child maltreatment as a risk factor for opioid dependence: Comparison of family characteristics and type and severity of child maltreatment with a matched control group. *Child Abuse & Neglect*, *33*, 343–352. doi:10.1016/j.chiabu.2008.09.009

Cooper, C. S. (2003). Drug courts: Current issues and future perspectives. *Substance Use & Misuse*, *38*, 1671–1711.

Dube, S. R., Anda, R. F., Whitfield, C. L., Brown, D. W., Felitti, V. J., Dong, M., & Giles, W. H. (2005). Long-term consequences of child sexual abuse by gender of victim. *American Journal of Preventive Medicine, 28*, 430–438.

Dvorak, R. D., Arens, A. M., Kuvaas, N. J., Williams, T. J., & Kilwein, T. M. (2013). Problematic alcohol use, trauma history, and PTSD symptom level: A path analysis. *Journal of Dual Diagnosis, 9*, 281–291. doi:10.1080/15504263.2013.835694

Elliott, D. E., Bjelajac, P., Fallot, R. D., Markoff, L. S., & Reed, B. G. (2005). Trauma-informed or trauma-denied: Principle and implementation of trauma-informed services for women. *Journal of Community Psychology, 33*, 461–477.

Fallot, R. D., & Harris, M. (2005). Integrated trauma services teams for women survivors with alcohol and other drug problems and co-occurring mental disorders. *Alcoholism Treatment Quarterly, 22*, 181–199.

Fallot, R. D., & Harris, M. (2006). *Trauma-informed services: A self-assessment and planning protocol*. Retrieved from http://www.annafoundation.org/TISA+PPROTOCOL.pdf

Falsetti, S. A., Resnick, H. S., Resick, P. A., & Kilpatrick, D. (1993). The Modified PTSD Symptom Scale: A brief self-report measure of posttraumatic stress disorder. *The Behavioral Therapist, 16*, 161–162.

Felitti, V. J. (2004). *The origins of addiction: Evidence from the adverse childhood experiences study*. Retrieved from http://www.acestudy.org/files/OriginsofAddiction.pdf

Gold, S. N. (2000). *Not trauma alone: Therapy for child abuse survivors in family and social context*. Philadelphia, PA: Brunner/Routledge.

Gold, S. N. (2002). Conceptualizing child sexual abuse in interpersonal context: Recovery of people, not memories. *Journal of Child Sexual Abuse, 10*, 51–71.

Holbrook, T. L., Galarneau, M. R., Dye, J. L., Quinn, K., & Dougherty, A. L. (2010). Morphine use after combat injury in Iraq and post-traumatic stress disorder. *New England Journal of Medicine, 362*, 110–117.

Hyman, S. M., Paliwal, P., Chaplin, T. M., Mazure, C. M., Rounsaville, B. J., & Sinha, R. (2008). Severity of childhood trauma is predictive of cocaine relapse outcomes in women but not men. *Drug and Alcohol Dependence, 92*, 208–216.

Kang, S., Magura, S., Laudet, A., & Whitney, S. (1999). Adverse effect of child abuse victimization among substance-using women in ireatment. *Journal of Interpersonal Violence, 14*, 657–670.

Klanecky, A. K., Harrington, J., & McChargue, D. E. (2008). Child sexual abuse, dissociation, and alcohol: Implications of chemical dissociation via blackouts among college women. *The American Journal of Drug and Alcohol Abuse, 34*, 277–284.

Marlowe, D. B. (2003). Integrating substance abuse treatment and criminal justice supervision. *Science and Practice Perspectives, 2*(1), 4–14.

McHugo, G. J., Caspi, Y., Kammerer, N., Mazelis, R., Jackson, E. W., Russell, L., . . . Kimerling, R. (2005). The assessment of trauma history in women with co-cccurring substance abuse and mental disorders and a history of interpersonal violence. *Journal of Behavioral Services & Research, 32*, 113–127.

Mills, K. L., Teesson, M., Ross, J., & Darke, S. (2007). The impact of post-traumatic stress disorder on treatment outcomes for heroin dependence. *Addiction, 102*, 447–454.

Mitchell, O., Wilson, D. B., Eggers, A., & MacKenzie, D. L. (2014). Assessing the effectiveness of drug courts on recidivism: A meta-analytic review of traditional and non-traditional drug courts. *Journal of Criminal Justice*, *40*(1), 60–71. doi:10.1080/15299732.2011.608781

Najavits, L. M., Gallop, R. J., & Weiss, R. D. (2006). Seeking safety therapy for adolescent girls with PTSD and substance use disorder: A randomized controlled trial. *Journal of Behavioral Health Services & Research*, *33*, 453–463.

Najavits, L. M., Schmitz, M., Gotthardt, S., & Weiss, R. D. (2005). Seeking safety plus exposure therapy: An outcome study on dual diagnosis men. *Journal of Psychoactive Drugs*, *27*, 425–435.

Najavits, L. M., & Walsh, M. (2012). Dissociation, PTSD, and substance abuse: An empirical study. *Journal of Trauma & Dissociation*, *13*(1), 115–126.

National Institute of Justice. (2012). *Drug courts*. Retrieved from http://www.nij.gov/topics/courts/drug-courts/

Nehls, N., & Sallmann, J. (2005). Women living with a history of physical and/or sexual abuse, substance use, and mental health problems. *Qualitative Health Research*, *15*, 365–381.

Ompad, D. C., Ikeda, R. M., Shah, N., Fuller, C. M., Bailey, S., Morse, E., . . . Strathdee, S. A. (2005). Childhood sexual abuse and age at initiation of injection drug use. *Research and Practice*, *95*, 703–709.

Ouimette, P. C., Kimerling, R., Shaw, J. & Moos, R. H. (2000). Physical and sexual abuse among women and men with substance use disorders. *Alcoholism Treatment Quarterly*, *18*, 7–17.

Pereda, N., Guilera, G., Forns, M., & Gomez-Benito, J. (2009). The prevalence of child sexual abuse in community and student samples: A meta-analysis. *Clinical Psychology Review*, *29*, 328–338.

Powell, C., Stevens, S., Lo Dolce, B., Sinclair, K. O., & Swenson-Smith, C. (2012). Outcomes of a trauma-informed Arizona family drug court. *Journal of Social Work Practice in the Addictions*, *12*, 219–241.

Putnam, F. W. (2003, March). Ten-year research update review: Child sexual abuse. *Journal of the American Academy of Child and Adolescent Psychiatry*, *42*, 269–278.

Rosen, C. S., Ouimette, P. C., Sheikh, J. L., Gregg, J. A., & Moos, R. H. (2002). Physical and sexual abuse history and addiction treatment outcomes. *Journal of Studies on Alcohol*, *63*, 683–687.

Sacks, J. Y., McKendrick, K., & Banks, S. (2008). The impact of early trauma and abuse on residential substance abuse treatment outcomes for women. *Journal of Substance Abuse Treatment*, *34*, 90–100.

Sartor, C. E., Lynskey, M. T., Bucholz, K. K., McCutcheon, V. V., Nelson, E. C., Waldron, M., & Heath, A. C. (2007). Childhood sexual abuse and the course of alcohol dependence development: Findings from a female twin sample. *Drug and Alcohol Dependence*, *89*, 139–144.

Sartor, C. E., McCutcheon, V. V., O'Leary, C. C., Van Buren, D. J., Allsworth, J. E., Jeffe, D. B., & Cottler, L. B. (2012). Lifetime trauma exposure and posttraumatic stress disorder in women sentenced to drug court. *Psychiatry Research*, *200*, 602–608.

Savage, A., Quiros, L., Dodd, S. J., & Bonavota, D. (2007). Building trauma informed practice: Appreciating the impact of trauma in the lives of women with substance abuse and mental health problems. *Journal of Social Work Practice in the Addictions*, *7*, 91–116.

Schumacher, J. A., Coffey, S. F., & Stasiewicz, P. R. (2006). Symptom severity, alcohol craving, and age of trauma onset in childhood and adolescent trauma survivors with comorbid alcohol dependence and posttraumatic stress disorder. *The American Journal on Addictions*, *15*, 422–425.

Siegel, J. A., & Williams, L. M. (2003). The relationship between child sexual abuse and female delinquency and crime: A prospective study. *Journal of Research in Crime and Delinquency*, *40*, 71–94. doi:10.1177/0022427802239254

Toussaint, D. W., VanDeMark, N. R., Bornemann, A., & Graeber, C. J. (2007). Modifications to the Trauma Recovery and Empowerment Model (TREM) for substance-abusing women with histories of violence: Outcomes and lessons learned at a Colorado substance abuse treatment center. *Journal of Community Psychology*, *35*, 879–894.

Turner, S., Longshore, D., Wenzel, S., Deschenes, E., Greenwood, P, Fain, T., . . . McBride, D. (2002). A decade of drug treatment court research. *Substance Use & Misuse*, *37*, 1489–1527.

Wiechelt, S. A., Miller, B. A., Smyth, N. J., & Maguin, E. (2011). Associations between post-traumatic stress disorder symptoms and alcohol and other drug problems: Implications for social work practice. *Practice: Social Work in Action*, *23*, 183–199. doi:10.1080/09503153.2011.597200

Zimmerman, M., & Mattia, J. I. (1999). The reliability and validity of a screening questionnaire for 13 DSM–IV Axis I disorders (the Psychiatric Diagnostic Screening Questionnaire) in psychiatric outpatients. *Journal of Clinical Psychiatry*, *60*, 677–683.

Zweig, J. M., Schlichter, K. A., & Burt, M. R. (2002). Assisting women victims of violence who experience multiple barriers to services. *Violence Against Women*, *8*, 162–180.

Factors Associated With Substance Use Disorders Among Traumatized Homeless Youth

SANNA J. THOMPSON, PhD
Associate Professor, School of Social Work, University of Texas at Austin, Austin, Texas, USA

KIMBERLY BENDER, PhD
Associate Professor, School of Social Work, University of Denver, Denver, Colorado, USA

KRISTIN M. FERGUSON, PhD
Associate Professor, Silberman School of Social Work, Hunter College, New York, New York, USA

YEONWOO KIM, MA
PhD Student, School of Social Work, University of Texas at Austin, Austin, Texas, USA

*This study aimed to identify homeless youths' lifestyle and trauma-related risk factors as well as protective factors associated with alcohol use disorder or no disorder and drug use disorder or no disorder. Youth receiving homeless services in Denver (*n = *201), Austin (*n = *200), and Los Angeles (*n = *200;* N = *601) completed quantitative interviews assessing demographic information, alcohol and drug use, homeless lifestyle risk factors, trauma-related risk factors, and protective factors. Findings showed differences in trauma-related risk factors between alcohol and drug use disorders, but not homeless lifestyle risks. Protective factors predicted substance use disorders beyond risk factors. Understanding trauma-related risk and protective factors associated with substance use disorders could improve interventions.*

Homeless youth are among this nation's most vulnerable populations. The McKinney–Vento Act (reauthorized in 2008) defines homeless youth as those who lack a fixed, regular, or adequate nighttime residence; these youth seek shelter in public places (e.g., parks, highway underpasses, abandoned buildings), share housing with others, live in emergency or transitional shelters, or have nighttime residences in places not designed for human sleeping accommodations. It has been estimated that 2.8 million youth (Hammer, Finkelhor, & Sedlak, 2002) are homeless in the United States and many use substances extensively (Baer, Peterson, & Wells, 2004).

Alcohol and drug use are consistently found to cooccur with trauma symptoms (Bender, Ferguson, Thompson, Komlo, & Pollio, 2010; Ginzler, Garrett, Baer, & Peterson, 2007); homeless youth who meet criteria for substance use disorders (SUDs) are three times more likely to have experienced a traumatic event than those without SUDs (Bender et al., 2010; Bender et al., 2012). Although SUDs are prominent among homeless youth and several factors have been found to be associated with serious use of substances, few studies have identified malleable protective factors that could inform services to prevent or reduce SUDs among homeless youth. Thus, the purpose of this study was to examine the extent to which protective factors buffer the effects of homeless lifestyle and trauma-related risk factors on homeless youths' SUDs.

SUBSTANCE USE DISORDERS

Rates of SUDs among homeless youth are two to three times higher than among their housed peers (Chen, Thrane, Whitbeck, & Johnson, 2006; Martijn & Sharpe, 2006); as many as 93% report experimenting with at least one illegal drug (Sussman et al., 1999; Thompson, Zittel-Palamara, & Forehand, 2005). Homeless youth are seven times more likely to use crack cocaine, five times more likely to use hallucinogens, and four times more likely to use heroin than housed peers (Slesnick, Meyers, Meade, & Segelken, 2000). Thus, it is clear that SUDs are a significant challenge among homeless youth.

HOMELESS LIFESTYLE RISK FACTORS FOR SUBSTANCE USE

Life on the street is characterized by extremely impoverished conditions and daily struggles to meet basic needs. Risk factors, defined as those intrapersonal and environmental factors that increase the likelihood of problem behaviors and negative outcomes (Fraser, Galinsky, & Richman, 1999; Fraser & Richman, 1999), include behaviors to attain limited resources. Most, if not all their needs are met through eating at soup kitchens, sleeping outdoors, and "spare-changing" (i.e., begging) for money (Roy, Haley, Boudreau, Leclerc, & Boivin, 2010). Youth engage in illegal (or marginally legal) income generation behaviors, such as prostitution or survival sex (i.e., participating in sexual acts in exchange for money, food, lodging, clothing, or drugs), pimping, pornography, theft, selling stolen goods, dealing drugs, or conning others for goods (Ferguson, Bender, Thompson, Xie, & Pollio, 2012; Halcón & Lifson, 2004; Whitbeck, Chen, Hoyt, Tyler, & Johnson, 2004). These behaviors are often viewed as necessary due to few formal employment opportunities, but might heighten the risk for substance use (Ferguson, Bender, et al., 2011; Taylor et al., 2008). The longer young people remain homeless, the more likely they are to engage in illegal income generation strategies and criminal behaviors, all of which are associated with substance use (Ferguson, Kim, & McCoy, 2011).

Among homeless youth identifying with a street lifestyle, abusing substances is viewed as a normative practice. Homeless young people report more favorable attitudes toward drug and alcohol use than their nonhomeless peers (Fors & Rojek, 1991). They use drugs and alcohol to help stay awake for extended periods, especially at night when the chances of victimization increase (Ayerst, 1999; Fest, 2003). Although maladaptive, substance use might allow homeless youth to repress or numb negative emotions (Kilpatrick et al., 2003) and escape from the stress associated with the dangers of street life or past trauma experiences (Thompson, 2005).

TRAUMA-RELATED RISK FACTORS FOR SUBSTANCE USE

Victimization and exposure to traumatizing events are part of the daily life of homeless young people. Homeless youth report being emotionally, physically, or sexually abused in their families before leaving home and this abuse is the primary reason given for running away (Tyler, Hoyt, & Whitbeck, 2000; Whitbeck, Hoyt, & Ackley, 1997). Once on the street, previous abuse might intensify the distress of street-related trauma experiences (Thompson, 2005; Ungar, 2013). Nearly 85% of homeless youth report various forms of trauma exposure and victimization while homeless (Stewart et al., 2004). In comparison to their housed peers, homeless youth experience disproportionately high rates of direct victimization, such as sexual assault, robbery, physical beating, and assault with a weapon (Tyler, Hoyt, Whitbeck, & Cauce, 2001). These youth also report experiences of indirect victimization, such as witnessing another person being sexually or physically assaulted, or overdosing on drugs (Stewart et al., 2004). Youth who experience direct or indirect victimization report higher rates of SUDs (Bender, Thompson, Ferguson, & Langenderfer, 2014).

Research suggests substance use, trauma exposure, and criminal behaviors are related (Wenzel, Andersen, Gifford, & Gelberg, 2001). Substance abuse amplifies deviant behaviors and might result in criminal behaviors and subsequent incarceration (Kipke, Simon, Montgomery, Unger, & Iversen, 1997). Criminal activity is typically associated with buying and selling drugs (Bender et al., 2012). On the other hand, high rates of exposure to violence and victimization increase homeless youths' use of substances to cope with life on the streets (Thompson, 2005). Some homeless youth report using substances to self-medicate and temporarily escape symptoms associated with trauma exposure (Bungay et al., 2006; Nyamathi et al., 2010). Termed *avoidance coping,* this maladaptive form of coping refers to strategies to avoid emotions and problems. Prior research suggests that the use of avoidant or disengagement coping strategies are associated with greater rates of both mental illness (e.g., depression) and behavior problems (Unger, Kipke, et al., 1998; Votta & Manion, 2003). Although drug use might provide a means of escape from the physical and emotional difficulties associated with surviving on the street (Zlotnick, Tam, & Robertson, 2003), this type of coping might provide initial relief but result in victimization (Bender et al., 2012).

PROTECTIVE FACTORS FOR SUBSTANCE USE

Although the stress of homelessness can increase the risk of SUDs, some homeless youth exhibit remarkable resiliency in managing a variety of stressors (Kidd, 2003; Rew & Horner, 2003). *Protective factors* refer to individual and environmental conditions that decrease the likelihood of problem behaviors or buffer the effects of risk (Fraser & Richman, 1999). One protective factor that has been shown to decrease the severity of substance abuse is generating income from legal sources, such as full-time, part-time, or temporary employment. One study found that homeless young adults who earned income from illegal sources were more likely to meet criteria for SUD, antisocial personality disorder, and major depression (Ferguson, Bender, & Thompson, 2014).

Homeless youths' healthy coping strategies appear protective. Problem-focused coping (i.e., attempts to address the problem or stressor directly) and social coping (i.e., use of social support to deal with stressors) might buffer the effects of risk. Extant research indicates that homeless youth who employed problem-focused coping strategies experienced positive health and mental health outcomes (Unger, Kipke, et al., 1998). Social coping, or drawing on peer supports (Kidd & Carroll, 2007), fulfills needs for love, companionship, and safety (Bender, Thompson, McManus, Lantry, & Flynn, 2007; Rew & Horner, 2003). Finally, youths' perspectives about their situations can be protective, as homeless youth view themselves as highly resilient, savvy to the street lifestyle, and independent (Rew, Taylor-Seehafer, Thomas, & Yockey, 2001). They believe that their feelings of personal competence and accepting themselves and their lives are expressions of resiliency (Rew et al.,

2001). Homeless youth who view themselves as optimistic describe their future as predictable, structured, and controllable (Heimberg, 1963). Those with greater positive expectations are less likely to be addicted to substances as compared to those with less positive expectations (Keough, Zimbardo, & Boyd, 1999). Thus, a more positive view of the future and feelings of resiliency might increase the likelihood that youth can capitalize on these strengths to survive street life (Bender et al., 2007) and overcome risks for SUDs.

Despite the high prevalence of SUDs among this population, limited research has examined risk and protective factors associated with alcohol and drug use disorders. Prior studies have largely adopted a lens of risk to identify predictors of substance abuse. This study challenges this perspective by also investigating protective factors that might provide malleable intervention targets aimed at preventing or treating homeless youths' SUD challenges. To assess the role both risk and protective factors play in understanding SUDs among homeless youth, this study posited the following research questions: Among homeless youth, what are the influences of homeless lifestyle risk factors (illegal income generation, arrest history, length of time homeless, transience), trauma-related risk factors (direct and indirect victimization on the street, childhood physical abuse or neglect, avoidance coping), and protective factors (legal income generation, social coping, problem-focused coping, personal competence, acceptance of self/life, optimism) on (a) alcohol abuse and dependency, and (b) drug abuse and dependency?

METHODS

Setting and Sample

A cross-sectional study was conducted with 601 youth (ages 18–24 years) receiving homeless youth services in Denver (n = 201), Austin (n = 200), and Los Angeles (n = 200). Agencies across the three cities were selected based on their existing relationships with researchers and their commitment to host the study. Multiservice, nonprofit organizations were recruitment sites, as they offered homeless, runaway, and at-risk young people a comprehensive system of care, including street outreach, meals, shelter, health care, counseling, and educational and employment services.

Using purposive sampling, street youth were recruited from homeless youth-serving agencies from March 2010 to April 2011. Recruitment procedures were nearly identical across the three cities with minor variations due to service offerings at each location (e.g., more crisis shelter users in Los Angeles, more drop-in service users in Denver and Austin). Inclusion criteria for youth participation in the study included (a) being 18 to 24 years of age, (b) being away from home for at least 2 weeks during the month prior to the interview, and (c) providing written informed consent. Agency case managers determined whether youth met these criteria and subsequently facilitated youth's introductions and referral to research staff. Participants were excluded if agency staff determined that they were incapable of comprehending the consent form due to cognitive limitations (psychotic symptoms or developmental delays). Youth who were noticeably intoxicated or high at the time of the interview were asked to return at a later time when they could more competently respond to interview questions. Agency staff determined youth eligibility for study recruitment based on their knowledge of each individual and their current level of intoxication. Although a refusal rate was not recorded across sites, very few youth refused to participate and the few that declined were typically unable to participate due to personal or service-oriented commitments at the time of the interview. Human subjects' approval was received at each investigator's university.

Once agency staff referred youth to research staff, study procedures were explained and written consent was obtained. Researchers administered a 45-minute quantitative retrospective interview containing both standardized self-report instruments and researcher-developed items that assessed a variety of issues, including demographic and background information, victimization experiences, substance use, and other factors. Interviewers read questions and response options aloud to participants who responded verbally. For one sensitive section of the survey focusing on childhood trauma, participants were given the option of reading and answering survey questions themselves. All interviews were conducted within the host agencies in private rooms. Participants were compensated with a $10 gift card to a local food vendor for their involvement in the quantitative interview.

Measures

Dependent variables

The SUD variables were determined using the Mini International Neuropsychiatric Interview (MINI; Sheehan et al., 1998). The MINI queries dichotomous (no–yes) screening and symptom questions for drug abuse and dependence and alcohol abuse and dependence during the past 12 months. Those who responded affirmatively to a prespecified number of symptoms were categorized as positive for alcohol abuse, alcohol dependence, drug abuse, or drug dependence (all coded 0 = *no,* 1 = *yes*; Lecrubier et al., 1997; Sheehan et al., 1998).

Demographics

Basic demographics included age, gender (0 = *male*, 1 = *female*), and ethnicity (1 = *White*, 2 = *Black*, 3 = *Hispanic*, 4 = *other*). Ethnicity was subsequently recoded as White = 1 and Black/Latino/other = 0. To assess and control for intercity differences, the city in which data were collected was also dummy coded (1 = *Los Angeles,* 2 = *Denver,* 3 = *Austin* [as reference group]). Youths' educational status was measured as 0 (*dropped out, suspended, or still enrolled in school*) or 1 (*graduated high school degree or General Educational Development [GED]*).

Homelessness Lifestyle Risk Factors

Transience was measured as the total number of times the youth had moved between cities since leaving home permanently. Responses were quantified by counting the number of cities (new or repeated) to which the youth had moved. Given the large skewness of the original variable (10.96), a log transformation was performed.

Length of time homeless was determined by subtracting the number of months since the youth had permanently left home from the interview date.

Arrest and incarceration history consisted of two variables. Arrest history was measured by asking participants the total numbers of time they had ever been arrested; incarceration history measured whether participants had ever been in jail (0 = *no,* 1 = *yes*).

Illegal income generation was derived from five questions that asked whether, during the past 6 months, the youth had gotten any resources to meet their basic needs from any one of five illegal (or legally regulated) sources: (a) panhandling, (b) dealing drugs, (c) survival sex (i.e., exchanging sexual acts for money, food, or lodging, or to meet other needs), (d) gambling, and (e) stealing (0 = *no,* 1 = *yes*). Responses to these five items were added to form a continuous variable that represented the number of illegal sources from which the young adults earned income during the prior 6 months (range = 0–5).

Trauma-Related Risk Factors

Childhood physical neglect and abuse variables were derived from the Childhood Trauma Questionnaire (CTQ; Bernstein, Ahluvalia, Pogge, & Handelsman, 1997). The CTQ is a 28-item retrospective self-report questionnaire designed to assess types of negative childhood experiences. This instrument has demonstrated reliability and validity, including test–retest reliability coefficients ranging from .79 to .86. *Physical abuse* included five CTQ items such as "I was punished with a belt, a board, a cord, or some other hard object." *Physical neglect* included five CTQ items such as "My parents were too drunk or high to take care of the family." Participants rated the truth of each statement on a scale ranging from 1 (*never true when they were growing up*) to 5 (*very often true when they were growing up*). For both physical abuse and neglect variables, whether or not participants had experienced any of the specific five types of abuse was dichotomized as 0 = *never true (no)* and 1 = *all else (yes)*.

Direct and indirect victimization on the streets consisted of two variables that were measured using a revised version of the Traumatic Life Events Questionnaire (Kubany et al., 2000), which assessed youths' frequency of experiencing different types of direct and indirect victimization while living on the streets. Items deemed most relevant for homeless youth were retained and less-relevant items were removed (e.g., natural disasters, warfare, or combat). Instructions asked youth to indicate how often they experienced various types of trauma, including physical assault by an acquaintance or a stranger, witnessing assault of another person, or being threatened with serious bodily harm. The response set included 0 = *never*, 1 = *once*, and 2 = *more than once*. Traumatic experiences were categorized as either *direct* (i.e., death of a friend or loved one, robbery, physical assault, sexual assault, and personal overdose) or *indirect* (i.e., received threats of death, witnessed severe assaults, or witnessed someone overdose), and then each was dichotomized to reflect 0 = *never experienced* and 1 = *experienced once or more*.

Avoidant-focused coping was measured by the Coping Scale (Kidd & Carroll, 2007), which identifies various means of coping. All items used a 5-point scale from 1 (*never*) to 5 (*almost always*) in response to the prompt "Please rate how much you use each of the following ways of dealing with problems." *Avoidant-focused coping* was assessed with two items (i.e., "Try not to think about it" and "Go to sleep"), which are coping strategies common among street youth (Carver, Scheier, & Weintraub, 1989). Responses were summed to form a continuous variable; higher scores represent higher levels of avoidant-focused coping (range = 0–10).

Protective Factors

Legal income generation was derived from seven questions that asked about methods used to generate income via legal or socially acceptable sources. Youth identified where they got any money or resources to meet their basic needs during the past 6 months from seven legal sources: (a) full-time employment, (b) part-time employment, (c) temporary paid employment, (d) selling self-made items, (e) selling bottles and cans, (f) selling clothing or other personal possessions, and (g) selling their blood or plasma (0 = *no*, 1 = *yes*). Responses were summed to form a continuous variable representing the number of legal sources from which the young people earned income during the previous 6 months (range = 0–7).

Problem-focused and social coping were two variables measured by the Coping Scale (Kidd & Carroll, 2007) to identify various positive means of coping. All items used a 5-point scale that was coded as 1 (*never*) to 5 (*almost always*) in response to the prompt "Please rate how much you use each of the following ways of dealing with problems." *Problem-focused coping* included two items ("Concentrated on what to do and how to solve the problem," and "Think about what happened and try to sort it out in my head"). *Social coping* was measured by one item that assessed how often the youth went to someone they trust for support. Derived from qualitative work by Kidd (2003), this method of coping is viewed as protective for dealing with experiences on the street.

Personal competence and acceptance of self/life consisted of two subscales from the Resilience Scale (Wagnild & Young, 1993). This scale includes 25 items that identify two major domains of resilience: (a) *personal competence* (self-reliance, independence, determination, invincibility, mastery, resourcefulness, and perseverance), and (b) *acceptance of self and life* (adaptability, balance, flexibility, and a balanced perspective of life). Participants rated their feelings on a scale from 1 (*strongly disagree*) to 7 (*strongly agree*); responses were summed to indicate higher scores reflect greater resiliency. The Resilience Scale has shown good to strong reliability, with alpha coefficients ranging from .72 to .94 (Rew et al., 2001; Wagnild, 2009).

Optimism, or feeling there was a positive future to look forward to, was measured by one subscale from the Future Time Perspective Scale (FTP; Heimberg, 1963). Each item on the FTP scale is scored from 1 (*strongly disagree*) to 7 (*strongly agree*), with higher scores indicating a more positive sense of the future. Five items for the optimism subscale include: "I have great faith in the future" and "I look forward to the future with hope and enthusiasm." Cronbach's alpha for this FTP subscale is strong ($\alpha = .71$).

Data Analysis

Global empirical analyses including means and standard deviations were used to describe youth's characteristics and demographics. Bivariate analyses using independent t tests and chi-square analyses examined significant relationships between independent variables (homeless lifestyle risk factors, trauma-related risk factors, and protective factors) and the dichotomous dependent variables (addicted or not addicted to alcohol and addicted or not addicted to drugs). To test for the likelihood of being in the category of addicted versus not addicted to alcohol or drugs, binary logistic regressions were computed. All independent variables significantly related to the dependent variable ($p \leq .05$) in bivariate analysis were entered into two separate hierarchical logistic regression models calculated with the full sample for (a) alcohol use disorder, and (b) drug use disorders. As risk and protective factors among homeless youth are interrelated and nonlinear, risk and protective factors were entered separately in blocks to test and separate the cumulative effects of risk and protective factors on SUDs. Correlates were entered in four blocks: Block 1 = demographics (age, gender, ethnicity, and education) and city of interview; Block 2 = Block 1 plus homeless lifestyle risk factors; Block 3 = Blocks 1 and 2 plus trauma-related risk factors; and

Block 4 = Blocks 1, 2, and 3 plus protective factors. The final hierarchical logical regression models for alcohol and drug use disorders highlight the cumulative effects of risk and protective factors on SUDs for alcohol and drugs separately.

RESULTS

Sample Demographics and Characteristics

Youth demographics across the three cities demonstrated that most participants were male (64.1%) and averaged 20 years of age (*SD* = 1.6). They were ethnically diverse, including youth who identified as White (39.9%), Black (25.3%), Latino (17.8%), and other ethnicities (17%). The majority had a high school education or GED (67.9%). On average, these youth had been homeless 2.7 years (*SD* = 2.6) and had moved on average 3.5 times (*SD* = 3.7) during the past year. In terms of alcohol abuse or dependency, nearly half (49.8%) met criteria for alcohol use disorder and 59.7% met criteria of drug use disorder during the past year. Approximately 20% of participants noted using no substances. Drugs that were commonly used by these youth included marijuana (76.7%), prescription drugs (34.8%), ecstasy (25.8%), cocaine (25.5%), hallucinogens (23.8%), over the counter drugs (19.3%), heroin or opiates (17.1%), methamphetamines (16%), and amphetamines (16%).

Youth characteristics varied depending on city of origin. For example, a greater proportion of youth in Los Angeles identified as Black (46%), whereas a greater proportion of youth in Austin identified as White (76%). More youth in Denver had completed high school or received their GED (83.1%) than did youth in the other cities. Austin youth were more transient (average of 5.8 moves), had been homeless longer (3.6 years), and were also the most likely to meet criteria for SUD for alcohol (70%) and drugs (74.5%) than youth from other cities. Due to these differences, city was a control variable in all analyses.

Alcohol Use Disorder

Bivariate results demonstrated significant differences between youth who met criteria for alcohol use disorder and those who did not, as shown in Table 1.

Table 2 displays the hierarchical logistic regression model predicting alcohol use disorder with each block of predictors (demographics, homeless lifestyle risk factors, trauma-related risk factors, and protective factors) entered sequentially. Specifically, demographics only accounted for 11% of the variance in alcohol use disorder, whereas the homeless lifestyle and trauma-related risk variables accounted for the most variance in alcohol use

TABLE 1 Alcohol and Drug Addiction Comparisons

	Alcohol addiction					Drug addiction				
	No alcohol addiction (n = 301)		Alcohol addiction (n = 299)			No drug addiction (n = 235)		Drug addiction (n = 359)		
	n M	% ±SD	n M	% ±SD	Chi-square or t test	n M	(%) ±SD	n M	(%) ±SD	Chi-square or t test
Demographics										
City					$\chi^2 = 50.3$***					$\chi^2 = 39.3$***
Los Angeles	119	19.8	81	13.4		108	18.0	92	15.3	
Denver	123	20.5	78	13.0		82	13.6	118	19.6	
Austin	59	0.10	140	23.3		45	7.5	149	25.0	
Age	19.9	±1.5	20.2	±1.7	$t = -2.6$*	20.0	±1.5	20.1	±1.7	$t = -.76$
Gender					$\chi^2 = 2.7$					$\chi^2 = 6.3$**
Male	183	60.8	201	67.2		136	57.9	244	68.0	
Female	118	39.2	98	32.8		99	42.1	115	32.0	
Ethnicity					$\chi^2 = 25.6$***					$\chi^2 = 20.1$***
White	210	69.8	150	50.3		67	28.5	168	46.9	
Other	91	30.2	148	49.7		168	71.5	190	53.1	
Education					$\chi^2 = 3.6$*					$\chi^2 = 1.9$
<High school	62	67.9	80	29.4		49	22.7	92	28.0	
HS graduate/GED	216	77.7	192	70.6		167	77.3	236	72.0	

Homeless lifestyle risk factors										
Transience (no. of moves)	2.4	±3.0	4.5	±4.0	$t = -7.3^{***}$	2.5	±3.1	4.1	±3.9	$t = -5.4$
Length homeless (months)	28.8	±29.4	36.1	±32.3	$t = -2.8^{**}$	30.4	±30.4	33.7	±31.4	$t = -1.4$
Total no. of arrests	3.86	±9.0	8.1	±13.1	$t = -4.6^{***}$	3.5	±9.3	7.5	±12.3	$t = -4.2^{***}$
Ever jailed	121	40.2	183	61.2	$\chi^2 = 2.5^{***}$	83	35.3	218	60.7	$\chi^2 = 36.7^{***}$
Illegal income generation	.36	±.68	.89	±.97	$t = -7.7^{***}$	.23	±.53	.88	±.97	$t = -9.3^{***}$
Trauma-related risk factors										
Childhood physical neglect	247	82.1	272	91.0	$\chi^2 = 10.2^{**}$	194	82.6	320	89.1	$\chi^2 = 5.3^{**}$
Childhood physical abuse	228	75.7	252	84.3	$\chi^2 = 6.8^{**}$	166	70.6	309	86.1	$\chi^2 = 21.1^{***}$
Direct street victimization	1.6	±1.5	2.5	±1.7	$t = -7.7^{***}$	1.4	±.09	1.7	±.09	$t = -7.6^{***}$
Indirect street victimization	1.2	±1.1	1.9	±1.1	$t = -9.0^{***}$	1.1	±1.1	1.8	±1.1	$t = -7.7^{***}$
Avoidant-focused coping	7.5	±2.7	9.2	±2.5	$t = -7.9^{***}$	7.3	±2.6	9.0	±2.6	$t = -7.9^{***}$
Protective factors										
Legal income generation	3.0	±1.7	3.9	±1.9	$t = -6.4^{***}$	2.9	±1.7	3.8	±1.9	$t = -5.7^{***}$
Problem-focused coping	7.9	±1.9	7.5	±1.8	$t = 2.4^{**}$	7.8	±2.0	7.6	±1.7	$t = 1.4$
Social coping	3.52	±1.3	3.06	±1.2	$t = 4.46^{***}$	3.53	±1.2	3.13	±1.2	$t = 3.84^{***}$
Personal competence	97.8	±13.7	94.7	±12.5	$t = 2.9^{**}$	98.1	±13.7	95.3	±12.1	$t = 2.7^{**}$
Acceptance of self/life	55.7	±8.7	54.7	±7.6	$t = 1.4$	55.8	±8.5	54.8	±7.8	$t = 1.4$
Optimism	20.3	±3.3	18.6	±3.5	$t = 9^{***}$	20.3	±3.2	18.9	±3.5	$t = 4.9^{***}$

Note. HS = high school; GED = general equivalency diploma.
$^{*}p \leq .05$. $^{**}p \leq .01$. $^{***}p \leq .001$.

TABLE 2 Alcohol Use Disorder Model

Youth characteristics	Model 1		Model 2		Model 3		Model 4	
	Exp(B)	CI	Exp(B)	CI	Exp(B)	CI	Exp(B)	CI
Demographics								
City (Austin reference)								
City (1): Los Angeles	.36***	[.21, .62]	.60	[.33, 1.06]	.69	[.37, 1.29]	.78	[.41, 1.50]
City (2): Denver	.31***	[.20, .50]	.42**	[.25, .72]	.39**	[.22, .70]	.44**	[.24, .80]
Age	1.02	[.90, 1.14]	1.05	[.92, 1.21]	1.05	[.90, 1.22]	1.05	[.90, 1.22]
Gender	1.25	[.86, 1.82]	.94	[.63, 1.41]	1.25	[.80, 1.97]	1.06	[.66, 1.71]
Ethnicity (White ref.)	1.33	[.88, 2.03]	1.14	[.72, 1.80]	1.31	[.80, 2.13]	1.39	[.84, 2.29]
HS graduate or Equivalent	.86	[.57, 1.30]	1.12	[.72, 1.76]	1.31	[.81, 2.12]	1.43	[.87, 2.35]
Homeless lifestyle risk factors								
Transience (no. of moves)			1.35**	[1.10, 1.65]	1.26*	[1.01, 1.56]	1.29*	[1.03, 1.62]
Length homeless (months)			1.00	[.99, 1.00]	.99	[.99, 1.00]	.99	[.99, 1.00]
Total number of arrests			1.02	[1.00, 1.04]	1.01	[.99, 1.04]	1.01	[.99, 1.04]
Ever jailed			1.55*	[1.01, 2.39]	1.16	[.73, 1.85]	1.27	[.79, 2.05]
Illegal income generation			1.89***	[1.48, 2.40]	1.40*	[1.08, 1.83]	1.27	[.96, 1.68]
Trauma-related risk factors								
Childhood physical neglect					1.64	[.87, 3.09]	1.68	[.87, 3.24]
Childhood physical abuse					.86	[.51, 1.45]	.85	[.50, 1.46]
Direct street victimization					1.17*	[1.01, 1.35]	1.16*	[1.00, 1.36]
Indirect street victimization					1.45**	[1.16, 1.80]	1.39**	[1.11, 1.75]
Avoidant-focused coping					1.21***	[1.12, 1.31]	1.21***	[1.11, 1.32]
Protective factors								
Legal income Generation							1.14*	[1.01, 1.29]
Problem-focused Coping							1.11	[.97, 1.26]
Social coping							.80*	[.67, .95]
Personal competence							.97*	[.94, 1.00]
Acceptance of self/life							1.05*	[1.01, 1.10]
Optimism							.95	[.89, 1.02]
Change-score statistics	$\chi^2(6, 548) = 50.995$, $p < .001$, adj. $R^2 = .118$		$\chi^2(11, 547) = 114.596$, $p < .001$, adj. $R^2 = .252$		$\chi^2(16, 543) = 168.847$, $p < .001$, adj. $R^2 = .356$		$\chi^2(22, 541) = 190.374$, $p < .001$, adj. $R^2 = .396$	

Note. HS = high school.
$^*p \leq .05$. $^{**}p \leq .01$. $^{***}p \leq .001$.

disorder (R^2 = .36). The fourth model with all predictor variables, including protective factors, was a significant improvement over previous models, indicating support for the cumulative effects of risk and protective factors on alcohol use disorder. In effect, the full model of risk and protective factors was significantly associated with homeless youths' alcohol use disorder (χ^2 = 190.37, p < .001) and resulted in a pseudo R^2 of .40.

The final model suggests differences in alcohol use disorder among the three cities; Austin youth were more likely to have alcohol use disorder than were youth from Denver (OR = .44, p < .01) but not significantly different than youth in Los Angeles. Of homeless lifestyle risk factors, youth who were more transient increased the likelihood for alcohol use disorder (OR = 1.29, p < .05). Among trauma-related risk factors, those who had been directly victimized on the street (OR = 1.16, p < .05) or indirectly victimized on the street (OR = 1.39, p < .01) were more likely to have alcohol use disorder, as were youth who utilized avoidant-focused coping (OR = 1.21, p < .001). Finally, regarding protective factors, using social coping strategies (OR = .80, p < .05), and possessing higher personal competence (OR = .97, p < .05) each decreased the likelihood of meeting diagnostic criteria for alcohol use disorder. Conversely, generating income from a greater variety of legal sources, such as formal employment (OR = 1.14, p < .05) and reporting a greater acceptance for oneself and life (OR = 1.05, p < .05) increased the likelihood of alcohol use disorder.

Drug Use Disorder

Similar to alcohol use disorder, Table 1 displays bivariate results indicating significant differences between those with drug use disorder and those with no drug use disorder. Hierarchical logistic regression analyses predicting drug use disorder followed the same analytic strategy used with alcohol use disorder (see Table 3). Similar to the alcohol use disorder model, each successive block significantly improved the model. Specifically, demographic variables accounted for 12% of the variance in drug use disorder. The additional homeless lifestyle risk factors increased the variance explained to 30% (R^2 = .30) and trauma-related risk variables also increased the variance explained (R^2 = .38). The fourth model that included demographic, risk, and protective factors was a significant improvement over previous models on drug use disorder (χ^2 = 199.40, p < .001, R^2 = .42).

Similar to the final model for alcohol use disorder, city differences were found; however, the likelihood for drug use disorder was less in Los Angeles (OR = .41, p < .05) compared to Austin, although Denver was not significantly different than Austin. Among homeless lifestyle risk factors, youth who had been homeless for a longer length of time were less likely to meet diagnostic criteria for drug use disorder (OR = 0.99, p < .05); whereas those who had ever been incarcerated (OR = 1.94, p < .01) or earned income

TABLE 3 Drug Use Disorder Model

	Model 1		Model 2		Model 3		Model 4	
Youth characteristics	Exp(B)	CI	Exp(B)	CI	Exp(B)	CI	Exp(B)	CI
Demographics								
City (Austin reference)								
City (1): Los Angeles	.24***	[.13, .42]	.37**	[.20, .68]	.40**	[.21, .78]	.41*	[.21, .81]
City (2): Denver	.43**	[.26, .71]	.59	[.33, 1.06]	.59	[.32, 1.11]	.64	[.33, 1.22]
Age	.91	[.81, 1.03]	.96	[.83, 1.11]	.94	[.81, 1.10]	.94	[.80, 1.10]
Gender	1.67**	[1.14, 2.43]	1.25	[.83, 1.90]	1.81*	[1.14, 2.86]	1.48	[.91, 2.42]
Ethnicity (White ref.)	1.22	[.78, 1.89]	1.02	[.63, 1.65]	1.22	[.72, 2.04]	1.24	[.73, 2.11]
HS grad or equivalent	.90	[.58, 1.38]	1.20	[.74, 1.93]	1.24	[.74, 2.07]	1.40	[.83, 2.38]
Homeless lifestyle risk factors								
Transience (no. of moves)			1.27*	[1.02, 1.58]	1.14	[.90, 1.44]	1.17	[.92, 1.49]
Length homeless (months)			.99	[.99, 1.00]	.99*	[.98, 1.00]	.99*	[.98, 1.00]
Total no. of arrests			1.01	[.99, 1.03]	1.01	[.99, 1.03]	1.01	[.98, 1.03]
Ever jailed			2.03**	[1.29, 3.20]	1.68*	[1.04, 2.74]	1.94**	[1.17, 3.20]
Illegal income generation			2.71***	[1.97, 3.72]	1.95***	[1.40, 2.72]	1.82***	[1.28, .2.59]
Trauma-related risk factors								
Childhood physical neglect					1.04	[.55, 1.97]	1.11	[.56, 2.18]
Childhood physical abuse					1.62	[.96, 2.74]	1.66	[.97, 2.85]
Direct street victimization					1.27**	[1.08, 1.49]	1.26**	[1.07, 1.48]
Indirect street victimization					1.13	[.90, 1.41]	1.09	[.86, 1.38]
Avoidant-focused coping					1.21***	[1.12, 1.32]	1.22***	[1.11, 1.33]
Protective factors								
Legal income generation							1.11	[.97, 1.26]
Problem-focused Coping							1.14	[.99, 1.31]
Social coping							.75**	[.62, .90]
Personal competence							.97*	[.94, 1.00]
Acceptance of self/life							1.06*	[1.01, 1.11]
Optimism							.98	[.90, 1.05]
Change-score statistics	$\chi^2(6, 542) = 49.828$, $p < .001$, adj. $R^2 = .119$		$\chi^2(11, 541) = 134.941$, $p < .001$, adj. $R^2 = .299$		$\chi^2(16, 537) = 179.540$, $p < .001$, adj. $R^2 = .384$		$\chi^2(22, 535) = 199.401$, $p < .001$, adj. $R^2 = .421$	

Note. HS = high school.
$^*p \leq .05$. $^{**}p \leq .01$. $^{***}p \leq .001$.

from a greater variety of illegal sources (OR = 1.82, $p < .001$) were more likely to meet criteria for drug use disorder. Regarding trauma-related risk factors, youth who had been directly victimized on the street (OR = 1.26, $p < .001$) or utilized avoidant-focused coping (OR = 1.22, $p < .001$) were more likely to have drug use disorder. Finally, among protective factors, using social coping strategies decreased the likelihood of meeting diagnostic criteria for drug use disorder (OR = .75, $p < .01$), as did having greater personal competence (OR = .97, $p < .05$). Higher scores on acceptance for oneself and life increased the likelihood that the participant met criteria of drug use disorder (OR = 1.06, $p < .01$).

DISCUSSION

This study examined homeless lifestyle and trauma-related risk factors as well as protective factors associated with SUDs among homeless youth. In this sample, the vast majority reported high levels of alcohol and drug use with more than half meeting criteria for alcohol or drug use disorders. These youth also used a wide variety of substances; the most commonly used drug was marijuana. These findings confirm previous research identifying high rates of addiction among this population (Thompson, 2005). Although rates of addiction were somewhat different across the three cities, they reflect the normative nature of substance use among this youth population (Peterson, Baer, Wells, Ginzler, & Garrett, 2006) and confirm that homeless youths' substance use goes beyond mere experimentation or occasional use.

As expected, a number of homeless lifestyle risk factors predicted alcohol and drug use disorder; however, risks diverged in terms of specific factors. For example, higher transience increased the likelihood of alcohol use disorder, but not drug use disorder. Youth who frequently move from place to place must constantly learn new environments and adapt to adversities related to securing shelter, food, social support, and formal resources (Bender et al., 2010). Thus, excessive use of alcohol might be a socialization method to fit in with other street youth in a new city or to cope with the stressors associated with moving to a new city. It is also likely that alcohol availability and access is greater than for drugs in new settings (Bender et al., 2010).

In contrast, no relationship was detected between transience and drug use disorder. Prior research on drug use disorder and transience among homeless youth could help explain this finding. One study found that homeless youth who met criteria for drug abuse and dependency were less likely to be transient, suggesting that drug-addicted youth choose to stay in one location versus moving frequently (Ferguson, Jun, Bender, Thompson, & Pollio, 2010). Whereas alcohol-addicted transient youth easily find access, youth with drug use disorder require a stable network to access their substance; thus, transience might disrupt this source. That transience was a predictor of alcohol use disorder but not drug use disorder suggests the differential impact of homeless risk factors on these youth and underscores the need for further research.

Conversely, length of time homeless; illegal or marginally legal methods of earning income such as panhandling, stealing, and drug distribution; and a history of incarceration were significant homeless lifestyle risk factors among those with drug use disorder, but not alcohol. The longer young people remain on the streets, the greater their entrenchment in the homeless lifestyle that is characterized by criminal activity, deviant peer groups, and substance use (Baron, 1999). Informal income generation, often termed *survival behavior*, is commonly used by homeless youth to subsist on the streets in the absence of legal or formal sources of income (Gaetz & O'Grady, 2002). However, these behaviors increase exposure to dangerous and criminal interactions with others (Ferguson et al., 2014). Youth who engage in drug distribution or prostitution are exposed to risk for assault and other types of victimization (Tyler & Beal, 2010), situations that lead to negative interactions with police, arrests, and even incarceration (Tucker, Edelen, Ellickson, & Klein, 2011). Taken together, these high-risk behaviors indicate youths' deeper involvement in illegal forms of survival strategies (Raleigh-DuRoff, 2004) that are likely to also encourage further entrenchment in the lifestyle of the street and SUDs (Thompson, Kim, Flynn, & Kim, 2007; Unger, Simon, et al., 1998).

With regard to trauma-focused risks, avoidant-focused coping was a significant risk factor for SUD. Avoidance behaviors, such as efforts to avert thoughts, feelings, conversations, or activities associated with the trauma are symptoms also experienced by traumatized individuals (Foa & Meadows, 1997). Substances blunt emotions to forget the stress and danger of street life, avoid thoughts of past traumatic experiences, and obscure distress (Bender et al., 2010; Ginzler et al., 2007). Although youth might experience immediate relief from using substances, it is a temporary solution resulting in increased risk and greater challenges for SUD (Bender et al., 2012). This finding suggests there is opportunity to replace such maladaptive coping with more effective coping methods by encouraging homeless youths to identify their stressors and devise strategies to address them, such as seeking supportive networks and building beliefs in their ability to change their lives and overcome current difficulties.

Most prominent among risk factors related to trauma were experiences of direct and indirect street victimization. Direct street victimization was a significant predictor of SUD for both alcohol and drugs, whereas indirect street victimization only predicted alcohol use disorder. These associations are collectively supported by research suggesting that direct experiences, such as assault and sexual victimization, as well as indirect experiences such as witnessing assault or being threatened, are associated with substance use disorder (Bender et al., 2012; Bender et al., 2014).

This study provides new insight into SUDs among homeless youth in that findings highlight malleable protective factors associated with decreased risk for alcohol or drug use disorders, even in the presence of significant lifestyle and trauma-related risks. Specifically, youth who reported greater personal competences and employed social coping methods were less likely to meet criteria for both alcohol and drug use disorders. This suggests that feeling competent to pursue a different way of life strengthens youths' self-efficacy and belief in their ability to succeed when faced with the adversities of homelessness and trauma. Social cognitive theory offers support for this finding in that greater self-efficacy and belief in one's abilities might improve coping skills needed to avert SUDs (Bandura, 1993).

Seeking help from supportive others might also help youth avoid SUD. This population often experiences social estrangement and isolation, especially among those with a greater time spent homeless (Baron, 2004). The lack of mentoring and monitoring by supportive peers, adults, and institutions increases the likelihood youth engage in risky behaviors, such as substance use (Osgood, Foster, & Courtney, 2010). Thus, connecting homeless youth with supportive adults and institutions, as well as prosocial peers, might reduce the likelihood of substance abuse or dependency. In one study, homeless youths who were connected to agency services reported a greater number of prosocial peers and fewer high-risk sexual and substance use behaviors than their counterparts who accessed agency services less frequently (Rice, Stein, & Milburn, 2008).

Unexpectedly, factors found to be protective in previous studies, namely legal income generation, increased the risk for alcohol, but not drug use disorder. Although further research is necessary to understand this association, Breslin and Adlaf (2005) found that among working adolescents, the greater number of hours worked per week, the higher their heavy episodic drinking. Similarly, Paschall, Ringwalt, and Flewelling (2002) suggested that the relationship between drinking and heavy alcohol use could be further explained by demographic characteristics. For example, age was positively associated with drinking and Black adolescents were less likely to report alcohol use than White youth. Although it is concerning that youth who generate income from legal and socially appropriate sources might abuse alcohol, it could be that homeless youth might simply have greater ability to purchase alcohol or have access to a larger network of coworkers and peers who also abuse alcohol.

Another purported protective factor, accepting oneself and one's life, also appears to be a risk factor for this sample of homeless youth, given that it increased the likelihood for SUDs for both alcohol and drugs. As homeless youth engage in normative street behaviors, such as substance use, that are supported by peers (Thompson et al., 2007; Unger, Simon, et al., 1998), they might feel it unnecessary to make changes and feel satisfied with their current situation. Homelessness encourages developing loose connections with similarly situated others to improve survival (Raleigh-DuRoff, 2004); these relationships might further encourage the self-perception that the status quo is acceptable, even desirable. That both legal income generation and acceptance of self and life were expected to be protective factors but were detected as risk factors in this study raises the question of whether the risk and resilience framework is overly simplistic for understanding SUDs among homeless youth.

Limitations

When interpreting these results, it is important to consider methodological limitations. First, this study's cross-sectional design cannot address the assumption of causal order. It is possible that risk and protective factors might not precede SUDs, but rather occur in tandem with the experiences of homelessness. Although challenging among this highly transient group of youth, future attempts using longitudinal data collection to better test these alternative explanations are needed. In addition, this study included a convenience sample of homeless young adults accessing services through homeless youth agencies in three cities. Although the sample might not be representative of homeless young adults across the United States, the basic demographics of the young people in this study appear similar to other studies of street-involved youth (Bousman et al., 2005; Rew, 2002). This study is also one of the first to assess substance use among those accessing homeless services in multiple geographic areas.

Social desirability might also be a concern due to the reliance on self-report measures. As participants were interviewed face-to-face at the agencies where they received services, it is possible that answers to sensitive questions, such as child maltreatment, illegal income generation, and street victimization, were answered in a way they perceived most desirable to the interviewer. In addition, the possibility of cultural bias could also be a factor, as homeless young people have a unique culture that identifies with a street "language" and expressing themselves counter to traditional authority (Bender et al., 2007). Interviewers were familiar with the homeless lifestyle and attempted to minimize these biases, but the fact that interviewers were "outsiders" might have influenced participant responses. However, interviewers found youth willing, even anxious, to describe their life experiences.

CONCLUSION

Despite the preceding limitations, this study has implications for service provision to homeless youth. The cluster of factors predicting alcohol and drug use disorders suggests that interventions must consider different dimensions of risk and protection related to homeless youth. Identifying youth with SUDs would help to allocate limited resources to those most at risk. Homeless youth with histories of victimization and substance use might be least likely to trust and engage formal and informal support systems (McManus & Thompson, 2008). In addition, SUDs might inhibit social-emotional skills (Gaetz, 2004) that impede youths' abilities to transition to more stable living situations. Thus, understanding trauma-related risk factors and protective factors associated with SUDs might provide guidance on methods to intervene and extend policies to address these specific issues (Bender et al., 2010; Stewart et al., 2004; Thompson, 2005).

REFERENCES

Ayerst, S. L. (1999). Depression and stress in street youth. *Adolescence, 34*, 567–575.

Baer, J. S., Peterson, P. L., & Wells, E. A. (2004). Rationale and design of a brief substance use intervention for homeless adolescents. *Addiction Research and Theory, 12*, 317–334.

Bandura, A. (1993). Perceived self-efficacy in cognitive development and functioning. *Educational Psychologist, 28*, 117–148.

Baron, S. W. (1999). Street youths and substance use: The role of background, street lifestyle, and economic factors. *Youth & Society, 31*(1), 3–26.

Baron, S. W. (2004). General strain, street youth and crime: A teset of Agnew's revised theoory. *Criminology, 42*, 457–484. doi:10.1111/j.1745-9125.2004.tb00526.x

Bender, K., Ferguson, K., Thompson, S., Komlo, C., & Pollio, D. (2010). Factors associated with trauma and posttraumatic stress disorder among homeless youth in three U.S. cities: The importance of transience. *Journal of Traumatic Stress, 23*(1), 161–168. doi:10.1002/jts.20501

Bender, K., Thompson, S. J., Ferguson, K., Komlo, C., Taylor, C., & Yoder, J. (2012). Substance use and victimization: Street-involved youths' perspectives and service implications. *Children and Youth Services Review, 34*, 2392–2399. doi: http://dx.doi.org/10.1016/j.childyouth.2012.09.008

Bender, K., Thompson, S., Ferguson, K., & Langenderfer, L. (2014). Substance use predictors of victimization profiles among homeless youth: A latent class analysis. *Journal of Adolescence, 37*, 155–164. doi:http://dx.doi.org/10.1016/j.adolescence.2013.11.007

Bender, K., Thompson, S. J., McManus, H., Lantry, J., & Flynn, P. M. (2007). Capacity for survival: Exploring strengths of homeless street youth. *Child Youth Care Forum, 36*, 25–42.

Bernstein, D. P., Ahluvalia, T., Pogge, D., & Handelsman, L. (1997). Validity of the Childhood Trauma Questionnaire in an adolescent psychiatric population. *Journal of the American Academy of Child & Adolescent Psychiatry, 36*, 340–348.

Bousman, C. A., Blumberg, E. J., Shillington, A. M., Hovell, M. F., Ji, M., Lehman, S., & Clapp, J. (2005). Predictors of substance use among homeless youth in San Diego. *Addictive Behaviors, 30*, 1100–1110.

Breslin, F. C., & Adlaf, E. M. (2005). Part-time work and adolescent heavy episodic drinking: The influence of family and community context. *Journal of Studies on Alcohol, 66*, 784–789.

Bungay, V., Malchy, L., Buxton, J. A., Johnson, J., Macpherson, D., & Rosenfeld, T. (2006). Life the jib: A snapshot of street youth's use of crystal methamphetamine. *Addiction Research and Theory, 14*, 235–251.

Carver, C. S., Reynolds, S. L., & Scheier, M. F. (1994). The Possible Selves of Optimists and Pessimists. *Journal of Research in Personality, 28*(2), 133–141.

Chen, X., Thrane, L., Whitbeck, L. B., & Johnson, K. (2006). Mental disorders, comorbidity, and post-runaway arrests among homeless and runaway adolescents. *Journal of Research on Adolescence, 16*, 379–402.

Ferguson, K., Bender, K., & Thompson, S. J. (2014). Social estrangement factors associated with income generation among homeless young adults in three U.S cities. *Journal for Society for Social Work and Research, 5*(4), 461–487.

Ferguson, F., Bender, K., Thompson, S. J., Maccio, E., Xie, B., & Pollio, D. (2011). Social control correlates of arrest behavior among homeless youth in five U.S. cities. *Violence and Victims, 26*, 648–668.

Ferguson, K. M., Bender, K., Thompson, S. J., Xie, B., & Pollio, D. (2012). Exploration of arrest activity among homeless young adults in four U.S. cities. *Social Work Research, 36*, 233–238. doi:10.1093/swr/svs023

Ferguson, K., Jun, J., Bender, K., Thompson, S., & Pollio, D. (2010). A comparison of addiction and transience among street youth: Los Angeles, California, Austin, Texas, and St. Louis, Missouri. *Community Mental Health Journal, 46*, 296–307.

Ferguson, K., Kim, M., & McCoy, S. (2011). Enhancing empowerment and leadership among homeless youth in agency and community settings: A grounded theory approach. *Child and Adolescent Social Work Journal, 28*(1), 1–22.

Fest, J. (2003). Understanding street culture: A prevention perspective. *School Nurse News, 20*(2), 16–18.

Foa, E., & Meadows, E. A. (1997). The psychosocial treatment for posttraumatic stress disorder: A critical review. *Annual Review of Psychology, 48*, 449–480.

Fors, S. W., & Rojek, D. G. (1991). A comparison of drug involvement between runaways and school youths. *Journal of Drug Education, 21*(1), 13–25.

Fraser, M. W., Galinsky, M. J., & Richman, J. M. (1999). Risk, protection, and resilience: Toward a conceptual framework for social work practice. *Social Work Research, 23*, 131–143. doi:10.1093/swr/23.3.131

Fraser, M. W., & Richman, J. M. (1999). Risk, production, and resilience: Toward a conceptual framework for social work practice. *Social Work Research, 23*, 131.

Gaetz, S. (2004). Safe streets for whom? Homeless youth, social exclusion, and criminal victimization. *Canadian Journal of Criminology and Criminal Justice, 46*, 423–455.

Gaetz, S., & O'Grady, B. (2002). Making money: Exploring the economy of young homeless workers. *Work, Employment and Society, 16*, 433–456.

Ginzler, J. A., Garrett, S. B., Baer, J. S., & Peterson, P. L. (2007). Measurement of negative consequences of substance use in street youth: An expanded use of the Rutgers Alcohol Problem Index. *Addictive Behaviors, 32*, 1519–1525.

Halcón, L. L., & Lifson, A. R. (2004). Prevalence and predictors of sexual risks among homeless youth. *Journal of Youth and Adolescence, 33*, 71–80.

Hammer, H., Finkelhor, D., & Sedlak, A. J. (2002). Runaway/throwaway children: National esitmates and characteristics. Washington, DC: U.S. Department of Justice, Office of Juvenile Justice and Delinquency Prevention.

Heimberg, L. K. (1963). *The measurement of future time perspective*. Nashville, TN: Vanderbilt University.

Keough, K. A., Zimbardo, P. G., & Boyd, J. N. (1999). Who's smoking, drinking, and using drugs? Time perspective as a predictor of substance use. *Basic and Applied Social Psychology, 21*, 149–164.

Kidd, S. A. (2003). Street youth: Coping interventions. *Child & Adolescent Social Work Journal, 20*, 235–261.

Kidd, S. A., & Carroll, M. R. (2007). Coping and suicidality among homeless youth. *Journal of Adolescence, 30*, 283–296.

Kilpatrick, D. G., Ruggiero, K. J., Acierno, R., Saunders, B. E., Resnick, H. S., & Best, C. L. (2003). Violence and risk of PTSD, major depression, substance abuse/dependence, and comorbidity: Results from the National Survey of Adolescents. *Journal of Consulting And Clinical Psychology, 71*, 692–700.

Kipke, M. D., Simon, T. R., Montgomery, S. B., Unger, J. B., & Iversen, E. F. (1997). Homeless youth and their exposure to and involvement in violence while living on the streets. *Journal of Adolescent Health, 20*, 360–367. doi:10.1016/S1054-139X(97)00037-2

Kubany, E. S., Haynes, S. N., Leisen, M. B., Owens, J. A., Kaplan, A. S., Watson, S. B., & Burns, K. (2000). Development and preliminary validation of a brief broad-spectrum measures of trauma exposure: The Traumatic Life Events Questionnaire. *Psychological Assessment, 12*, 210–224.

Lecrubier, Y., Sheehan, D., Weiller, E., Amorim, P., Bonora, I., Sheehan, K., . . . Dunbar, G. (1997). The MINI International Neuropsychiatric Interview—A short diagnostic structured interview: Reliability and validity according to the CIDI. *European Psychiatry, 12*, 224–231.

Martijn, C., & Sharpe, L. (2006). Pathways to youth homelessness. *Social Science & Medicine, 62*(1), 1–12.

McManus, H. H., & Thompson, S. J. (2008). Trauma among unaccompanied homeless youth: The integration of street culture into a model of intervention. *Journal of Aggression, Maltreament & Trauma, 16*, 92–109. doi:10.1080/10926770801920818

Nyamathi, A., Hudson, A., Greengold, B., Slagle, A., Marfisee, M., Khalilifard, F., & Leake, B. (2010). Correlates of substance use severity among homeless youth. *Journal of Child & Adolescent Psychiatric Nursing, 23*, 214–222. doi:10.1111/j.1744-6171.2010.00247.x

Osgood, D. W., Foster, E. M., & Courtney, M. E. (2010). Vulnerable populations and the transition to adulthood. *Future Child, 20*, 209–229.

Paschall, M. J., Ringwalt, C. L., & Flewelling, R. L. (2002). Explaining higher levels of alcohol use among working adolescents: An analysis of potential explanatory variables. *Journal of Studies on Alcohol, 63*, 169–178.

Peterson, P. L., Baer, J. S., Wells, E. A., Ginzler, J. A., & Garrett, S. B. (2006). Short-term effects of a brief motivational intervention to reduce alcohol and drug risk among homeless adolescents. *Psychology of Addictive Behaviors, 20*, 254–264.

Raleigh-DuRoff, C. (2004). Factors that influence homeless adolescents to leave or stay living on the street. *Child & Adolescent Social Work Journal*, *21*, 561–571.

Rew, L. (2002). Characteristics and health care needs of homeless adolescents. *Nursing Clinics of North America*, *37*, 423–431.

Rew, L., & Horner, S. D. (2003). Personal strengths of homeless adolescents living in a high-risk environment. *Advances in Nursing Science*, *26*, 90–101.

Rew, L., Taylor-Seehafer, M., Thomas, N. Y., & Yockey, R. D. (2001). Correlates of resilience in homeless adolescents. *Journal of Nursing Scholarship*, *33*(1), 33–40.

Rice, E., Stein, J. A., & Milburn, N. (2008). Countervailing social network influences on problem behaviors among homeless youth. *Journal of Adolescence*, *31*, 625–639. doi:10.1016/j.adolescence.2007.10.008

Roy, E., Haley, N., Boudreau, J. F., Leclerc, P., & Boivin, J. F. (2010). The challenge of understanding mortality changes among street youth. *Journal of Urban Health*, *87*(1), 95–101. doi:10.1007/s11524-009-9397-9

Sheehan, D. V., Lecrubier, Y., Sheehan, K. H., Amorim, P., Janavs, J., Weiller, E., . . . Dunbar, G. C. (1998). The Mini-International Neuropsychiatric Interview (M.I.N.I.): The development and validation of a structured diagnostic psychiatric interview for DSM–IV and ICD–10. *Journal of Clinical Psychiatry*, *59*(Suppl. 20), 22–33.

Slesnick, N., Meyers, R. J., Meade, C. S., & Segelken, D. H. (2000). Bleak and hopeless no more: Treatment engagement of substance abusing runaway youth and their families. *Journal of Substance Abuse Treatment*, *19*, 215–222.

Stewart, A. J., Steiman, M., Cauce, A. M., Cochran, B. N., Whitbeck, L. B., & Hoyt, D. R. (2004). Victimization and posttraumatic stress disorder among homeless adolescents. *Journal of American Academy of Child & Adolescent Psychiatry*, *43*, 325–331. doi:10.1097/00004583-200403000-00015

Sussman, S., Simon, T. R., Stacy, A. W., Dent, C. W., Ritt, A., Kipke, M. D., . . . Flay, B. R. (1999). The association of group self-identification and adolescent drug use in three samples varying in risk. *Journal of Applied Social Psychology*, *29*, 1555–1581.

Taylor, C. A., Boris, N. W., Heller, S. S., Clum, G. A., Rice, J. C., & Zeanah, C. H. (2008). Cumulative experiences of violence among high-risk urban youth. *Journal of Interpersonal Violence*, *23*, 1618–1635. doi:10.1177/0886260508314323

Thompson, S. J. (2004). Risk/protective factors associated with substance use among runaway/homeless youth utilizing emergency shelter services nationwide. *Substance Abuse*, *25*(3), 13–26.

Thompson, S. J. (2005). Factors associated with rauma symptoms among runaway/homeless adolescents. *Stress, Trauma, and Crisis*, *8*, 143–156. doi:10.1080/15434610590956912

Thompson, S. J., Kim, J., Flynn, P., & Kim, H. (2007). Peer relationships: Comparison of homeless youth in the U.S. and South Korea. *International Social Work*, *50*, 783–795.

Thompson, S. J., Zittel-Palamara, K., & Forehand, G. (2005). Difference in risk factors for cigarette, alcohol, and marijuana use among runaway youth utilizing two services sectors. *Journal of Child & Adolescent Substance Abuse*, *15*(1), 17–36.

Tucker, J., Edelen, M., Ellickson, P., & Klein, D. (2011). Running away from home: A longitudinal study of adolescent risk factors and young adult outcomes. *Journal of Youth and Adolescence*, *40*, 507–518.

Tyler, K. A., & Beal, M. R. (2010). The high-risk environment of homeless young adults: Consequences for physical and sexual victimization. *Violence & Victims*, *25*(1), 101–115.

Tyler, K. A., Hoyt, D. R., & Whitbeck, L. B. (2000). The effects of early sexual abuse on later sexual victimization among female homeless and runaway adolescents. *Journal of Interpersonal Violence*, *15*, 235–250.

Tyler, K. A., Hoyt, D. R., Whitbeck, L. B., & Cauce, A. M. (2001). The impact of childhood sexual abuse on later sexual victimization among runaway youth. *Journal of Research on Adolescence*, *11*, 151.

Ungar, M. (2013). Resilience, trauma, context, and culture. *Trauma, Violence, & Abuse*, *14*, 255–266. doi:10.1177/1524838013487805

Unger, J. B., Kipke, M. D., Simon, T. R., Johnson, C. J., Montgomery, S. B., & Iverson, E. (1998). Stress, coping, and social support among homeless youth. *Journal of Adolescent Research*, *13*, 134–157. doi:10.1177/0743554898132003

Unger, J. B., Simon, T. R., Newman, T. L., Montgomery, S. B., Kipke, M. D., & Albornoz, M. (1998). Early adolescent street youth: An overlooked population with unique problems and service needs. *Journal of Early Adolescence*, *18*, 325–348.

Votta, E., & Manion, I. G. (2003). Factors in the psychological adjustment of homeless adolescent males: The role of coping style. *Journal of American Academy of Child and Adolescent Psychiatry*, *42*, 778–785.

Wagnild, G. (2009). A review of the Resilience Scale. *Journal of Nursing Measurement*, *17*(2), 105–113.

Wagnild, G., & Young, H. (1993). Development and psychometric evaluation of the Resilience Scale. *Journal of Nursing Measurement*, *1*(2), 165–178.

Wenzel, S. L., Andersen, R. M., Gifford, D. S., & Gelberg, L. (2001). Homeless women's gynecological symptoms and use of medical care. *Journal of Health Care to Poor and Underserved*, *12*, 323–341.

Whitbeck, L. B., Chen, X., Hoyt, D. R., Tyler, K. A., & Johnson, K. D. (2004). Mental disorder, subsistence strategies, and victimization among gay, lesbian, and bisexual homeless and runaway adolescents. *Journal of Sex Research*, *41*, 329–342. doi:10.1080/00224490409552240

Whitbeck, L. B., Hoyt, D. R., & Ackley, K. A. (1997). Abusive family backgrounds and later victimization among runaway and homeless adolescents. *Journal of Research on Adolescence*, *7*, 375–392.

Zlotnick, C., Tam, T., & Robertson, M. J. (2003). Disaffiliation, substance use, and exiting homelessness. *Substance Use & Misuse*, *38*, 577–599.

Traumatic Experiences and Drug Use by LGB Adolescents: A Critical Review of Minority Stress

JEREMY GOLDBACH, PhD
Assistant Professor, School of Social Work, University of Southern California, Los Angeles, California, USA

BENJAMIN W. FISHER, MA
PhD Student, Peabody Research Institute, Vanderbilt University, Nashville, Tennessee, USA

SHANNON DUNLAP, MSW
PhD Student, School of Public Affairs, University of California, Los Angeles, Los Angeles, California, USA

High rates of illicit drug use found among lesbian, gay, and bisexual (LGB) adolescents are often attributed to unique and chronic traumatic events tied to sexual minority identity. Although initiation of drug use is relatively common within adolescence, little research contributes to our understanding of the disparities found among LGB adolescents. This review synthesized existing literature to determine if the minority stress model is applicable to LGB drug use disparities and fits within a trauma framework. Findings indicate that minority stress experiences have been inconsistently related to drug use among LGB adolescents. Implications for future research and practice are described.

Lesbian, gay, and bisexual (LGB) adolescents report significantly higher rates of drug use when compared to their heterosexual counterparts (Marshal et al., 2008; Moon, Fornili, & O'Briant, 2007; Remafedi, 1987), including use of marijuana and other illicit substances (Bontempo & D'Augelli, 2002; Corliss et al., 2010; Russell, Driscoll, & Truong, 2002). LGB adolescents are more likely to engage in polydrug use and report both higher rates of early drug use and a more rapidly increasing trajectory of use into adulthood when compared to their heterosexual peers (Garofalo, Wolf, Kessel, Palfrey, & DuRant, 1998; Marshal, Friedman, Stall, & Thompson, 2009).

Minority stress theory (Hatzenbuehler, Pachankis, & Wolff, 2012; Meyer, 2003) suggests that there are unique and traumatic experiences specific to identification as a sexual minority that result in a myriad of negative behavioral health outcomes. The extant literature proposes a number of criteria to define a traumatic event (Goodman, Corcoran, Turner, Yuan, & Green, 1998; Rowell & Thomley, 2013). A traumatic event might be sudden and unexpected but not lead to physical injury (Rowell & Thomley, 2013), could be cumulative (Follette, Polusny, Bechtle, & Naugle, 1996), and could include non-life-threatening or noncatastrophic events such as bullying, racism, or separation from family (Alessi, Meyer, & Martin, 2013). Epidemiological studies among adults have supported this framework, finding that sexual minorities report more pervasive and traumatic experiences in comparison to heterosexuals. For example, individuals who report having same-sex sexual partners at some point in their lifetime have a greater risk of child maltreatment, interpersonal violence, intimate partner violence, sexual assault (Balsam, Rothblum, & Beauchaine, 2005), child abuse or neglect (Alvy, Hughes, Kristjanson, & Wilsnack, 2013), hate crimes (Herek, 2009), trauma to a close friend or relative, and unexpected death of close family members when compared to heterosexuals (Roberts, Austin, Corliss, Vandermorris, & Koenen, 2010).

For LGB adolescents, traumatic events could also take the form of stress around disclosing to family and peers and expectations of their reactions, particularly as subsequent homelessness is not an uncommon outcome (Almeida, Johnson, Corliss, Molnar, & Azreal, 2009; Grossman et al., 2009; Haas et al., 2010; Remafedi, 1987). In-school victimization or bullying is also an increasing concern (Bailey & Phariss, 1996; Russell, Ryan, Toomey, Diaz, & Sanchez, 2011; Toomey, Ryan, Diaz, & Russell, 2011). Gay males are 8 times more likely and lesbian females 10 times more likely to experience victimization when compared to their heterosexual peers (D'Augelli & Grossman 2001; Kosciw, Palmer, Kull, & Greytak, 2013).

Given the significant public health impact of drug use, interventions to prevent the onset and delay progression are a priority for the Substance Abuse and Mental Health Services Administration (SAMHSA) and the Centers for Disease Control and Prevention (CDC). Further, both Healthy People 2020 and SAMHSA (U.S. Department of Health and Human Services,

Healthy People 2020, 2011; U.S. Department of Health and Human Services, Substance Abuse and Mental Health Services Administration, 2011) have identified a need for providing culturally appropriate services to sexual minority persons. An important first step in the development of targeted drug use interventions for LGB adolescents is a clearer understanding of how minority-specific traumatic events are relevant to their drug use (Goldbach & Holleran Steiker, 2011; Goldbach, Tanner-Smith, Bagwell, & Dunlap, 2014). From identified factors, targeted interventions can be developed that result in changes in use patterns, as have been done in studies of racial and ethnic minority youth (Cervantes & Goldbach, 2012). To aid in the development of prevention programming, this review follows Preferred Reporting Items for Systematic Reviews and Meta-Analyses (PRISMA) standards for systematic review in an effort to synthesize the extant literature on minority stress-related correlates of drug use among LGB adolescents. Given that alcohol use is both common among all adolescents and its use has been declining over the past two decades (National Institute on Drug Abuse, 2008), we focus this review on the use of other illicit substances in an effort to better target prevention efforts.

METHODS

Data Sources

We conducted a systematic search for both peer-reviewed and unpublished reports examining the relationship between LGB-related stressors and drug use in LGB youth using the best practices for systematic reviews as outlined in the Preferred Reporting Items for Systematic Reviews and Meta-Analyses (PRISMA; Moher, Liberati, Tetzlaff, Altman, & The PRISMA Group, 2009). PRISMA provides evidence-based guidelines for conducting and reporting systematic reviews, and our methods closely adhered to these guidelines. In our initial electronic search, we used the following electronic databases to find relevant reports: PsycINFO, PubMED, EBSCO, and ProQuest Dissertations & Theses. Two authors searched report titles, abstracts and subject lines using the terms "gay," "lesbian," "bisexual," or "sexual minority" paired with "youth" or "adolescent" and "drug use" or "substance abuse." Additionally, an ancestral approach (White, 1994) was used, where the citation lists of reports that met inclusion criteria were reviewed for additional research that might not have been identified through the electronic method. The electronic search process was replicated four times between August 2011 and September 2013.

Inclusion Criteria

To determine the scope of this review, we established eligibility criteria a priori that guided which reports would be eligible for inclusion as recommended in the PRISMA guidelines. Reports that did not meet all of the eligibility criteria were excluded from our analyses. Because we included both qualitative and quantitative reports in this review, we had to slightly alter some of our eligibility criteria depending on the methods used. Two authors reviewed each report to ensure its eligibility for inclusion in this study. Those alterations are noted in what follows. We made our eligibility decisions according to the following criteria.

Participants

To be included in this review, study participants initially needed to be (a) between the ages of 12 and 18, the general years of middle and high school (although enrollment in school was not a criterion for eligibility); and (b) identify as a sexual minority (lesbian, gay, or bisexual). Studies with participants who had a wider age range were ultimately included for analysis as almost all studies included broader age ranges. Thus, we ultimately included studies if participants were either (a) under age 18; or (b) were retrospectively reporting on their adolescence (e.g., Russell et al., 2011). This challenge to adolescent-specific research with LGB youth is described elsewhere in the literature (Elze, 2007). Additionally, studies that included both LGB and non-LGB youth were included if the author(s) conducted a subgroup analysis on the portion of the sample that identified as lesbian, gay, or bisexual. Unless participants were defined as "gay," we did not include literature on participants only described as men who have sex with men (e.g., Clatts, Goldsamt, Huso, & Gwadz, 2005) as this term focuses on behavior rather than identity, and we were particularly interested in youth who identify as lesbian, gay, or bisexual. As Young and Meyer (2005) argued, "*MSM* . . . [implies] absence of community, social networks, and relationships in which same-gender pairing is shared and supported" (p. 1145). Studies with multiple time points were included if the first time point occurred during adolescence.

Study Design

Extending a previous meta-analysis that explored relationship between minority stress and drug use among LGB adolescents (Goldbach et al., 2014), this systematic review included both qualitative and quantitative reports in the final analysis along with unpublished works such as dissertations. For quantitative reports, we included any study that examined the relationship between LGB-related minority stressors and drug use, including both cross-sectional and longitudinal designs. For qualitative reports, we relied on the original authors' analysis and interpretation of findings, where they stated an apparent relationship (or lack of relationship) between the LGB-related stress factor and the drug use pattern.

Comparison

Because we were interested in the role that the presence of minority stress factors would play on drug use, we included reports that explored differences within samples of LGB participants and did not include reports that only compared substance abuse outcomes between LGB and heterosexual samples (see Marshal et al., 2008; Marshal, et al., 2009, for a thorough analysis of this topic). Additionally, reports that included only the prevalence of drug use in LGB adolescents were not included, as these fell outside the scope of this review.

Variables of Interest

Eligible reports measured the relationship between a minority stressor related to participants' status as lesbian, gay, or bisexual and an illicit drug use outcome (not alcohol). For the purposes of this analysis, minority stressors were defined as perceived negative thoughts, feelings, or experiences that occurred because of one's sexual orientation. We excluded reports that only mentioned stressors that were unrelated to sexual orientation. In the qualitative reports, we relied on participants' words and authors' interpretations to identify the presence and impact of LGB-related minority stressors. Examples of LGB-related minority stressors include but are not limited to peer victimization, being kicked out of the home, and feeling rejected because of one's sexual orientation. Eligible drug use measures included those of recent or lifetime use of illicit substances such as marijuana, cocaine, heroin, and prescription pills.

Setting

We included reports in this review if they reported on research conducted in the United States. Also, to include only contemporary perspectives, we included reports published after January, 1990 to the present date (December 2013).

Data Collection and Analysis

Once eligible reports were identified, two coders independently read each report and coded for the following variables: quantitative, qualitative, or mixed methods; total sample size; percent of the sample that identified as a sexual minority; age range, mean, and standard deviation; sampling strategy; data collection process; minority stressor; measure of drug use; and relationship between minority stressor and drug use. Any discrepancies in coding were handled by bringing in a third coder and coming to consensus among those three.

Two members of the research team independently reviewed the included reports and organized the minority stressors into preliminary categories. On completion, reviewers met to achieve consensus and determine a final set of categories. Only minor variations were discovered between the two reviewers, which influenced the findings minimally. For example, one reviewer identified depression and psychological distress as separate categories, whereas the other reviewer only identified psychological distress; after discussion, the two separate categories were collapsed into a single one because depression is subsumed in the category of psychological distress. Because the data for this study came from both quantitative and qualitative studies that used a wide range of methods, we did not attempt to extract an overall "effect" of any given minority stressor on drug use outcomes. Rather, we summarized the relationship between each minority stress category and the corresponding substance abuse outcomes and noted patterns of both consistency and inconsistency within each category.

To assess the risk of bias within each study, we coded for the sampling method used. Because sexual minority youth are a vulnerable population and more difficult to sample, we expected many of the studies to use convenience sampling strategies, therefore limiting the generalizability of the original studies' findings as well as those of our systematic review. Moreover, we are aware of the potential of a systematic bias across studies where respondents might be withholding in their responses, possibly because of their perceived vulnerability and stigma. We were unable to formally measure this, but did hold it in mind when reporting and interpreting our findings. Additionally, we tried to guard against publication bias by including unpublished dissertations and theses.

RESULTS

We identified a total of 801 articles via our initial search of electronic databases and the citations of eligible reports. As displayed in Figure 1, our eligibility criteria led us to retain 24 of these studies for our review.

Each eligible report explored the relationship between an LGB-specific risk factor and drug use by LGB adolescents. Descriptive statistics of eligible reports such as sample characteristics and major study findings can be found in Table 1.

We organized the eligible reports into thematic categories related to psychological distress (8), family support and rejection (7), social support (5), housing instability (3), victimization (10), and questioning identity (1). Several reports addressed multiple minority stress factors and are listed separately. The major findings and patterns of results found across the 24 reports are described in Table 1. We found a diversity of geographic locations among the studies (Massachusetts, Vermont, New York, Washington, DC,

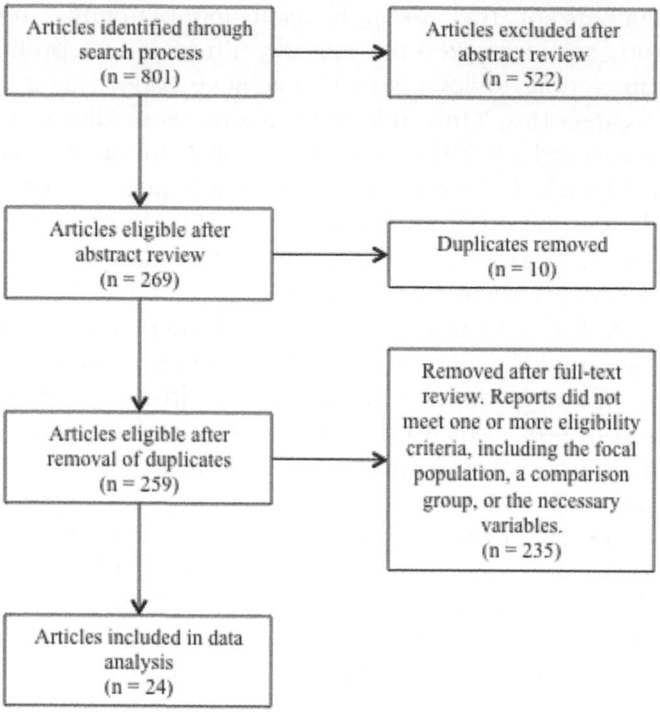

FIGURE 1 Flow chart of primary study inclusion.

Pennsylvania, Indiana, California, New Hampshire, Pennsylvania, Indiana, and three "Midwestern cities").

Psychological Distress

A commonly discussed correlate of drug use in the literature was the experience of psychological distress related to LGB identity. Specifically, this included measures of internalized homophobia (Gaddis, 2011; Gilmore, 1996; Rosario, Schrimshaw, & Hunter, 2008; Willoughby, Doty, & Malik, 2010), distress around coming out (Padilla, Crisp, & Rew, 2010; Rosario, Schrimshaw, & Hunter, 2009; Rosario, Rotheram-Borus, & Reid, 1996), general distress (Rosario, Hunter, & Gwadz, 1997; Savin-Williams & Ream, 2003; Wright & Perry, 2006) and "gay-specific" distress (Gilmore, 1996; Rosario et al., 2008), each of which was associated with increased drug use among LGB youth.

Several reports indicated that the coming out process often represented a time of increased interpersonal and intrapersonal distress (Pilkington & D'Augelli, 1995; Ryan, Huebner, Diaz, & Sanchez, 2009; Rosario et al., 2009). During this time, many LGB youth use substances to enhance social confidence and mitigate the distress associated with navigating a new identity (Hughes & Eliason, 2002). These reports indicated that it was not the number

TABLE 1 Table of Included Articles

Stressors and author	Sample characteristics: N	Age range	M age	SD	% LGB	Sample strategy	Data collection strategy	Substance use measure	Key findings: IV–DV relationship
Psychological distress									
Rosario, Rotheram-Borus, & Reid (1996)	136	14–19	16.8	1.4	100%	Convenience	In-person interviews; quantitative	Drug and Alcohol Survey for Adolescents to assess drug use frequency over past 3 months using a 3-point response scale	Parents discovering LGB identity, other kin discovering LGB identity, and being ridiculed by others were related to increased drug use within last 3 months.
*Rosario, Hunter, & Gwadz (1997)	154	14–21	18.3	1.6	100%	Convenience	In-person interviews; quantitative	Lifetime, past 3-month use, age of initiation of use, and lifetime frequency of use of a series of specific substances; frequency of heavy use was also assessed	As psychological distress increased, substance use increased.
*Rosario, Schrimshaw, & Hunter (2009)	156	14–21	18.3	1.6	5%	Convenience	In-person interviews; quantitative	Frequency of marijuana use in past 3 and 6 months; how many joints they usually smoke when they use marijuana	Negative reactions to disclosure of sexual orientation was associated with increased marijuana use, but positive/neutral reactions were not.
Gilmore (1996)	105	14–21	18	—	100%	Convenience	Paper surveys; quantitative	Scale score for substance abuse made up of items assessing frequency of use of various drugs	Increased stress associated with increased substance use. LGB-related stress not associated with substance use. Depression was also correlated with increased substance use.
Gaddis (2011)	12	45–62	Not reported	Not reported	100%	Convenience sample	Semistructured interview; qualitative	Qualitative discussion of substance use	Denial of lesbian identity was associated with substance use for coping at a young age.

(*Continued*)

TABLE 1 (Continued)

Stressors and author	Sample characteristics					Sample strategy	Data collection strategy	Substance use measure	Key findings: IV–DV relationship
	N	Age range	M age	SD	% LGB				
*Padilla, Crisp, & Rew (2010)	1906	12–17	16	—	100% (54.56% gay, 10.81% lesbian, 34.63% bisexual)	National convenience sample	Online surveys; quantitative	Dichotomous variable: use of marijuana, cocaine, ecstasy, or crystal meth in past 30 days	Higher likelihood of substance use among youth who had disclosure stress
*Rosario, Schrimshaw, & Hunter (2008)	76	14–21	Not reported	Not reported	100% women	Convenience	In-person interviews; quantitative	Frequency of marijuana use in past 3 and 6 months; how many joints they usually smoke when they use marijuana	Higher levels of LGB-related stress and internalized homophobia correlated with higher levels of marijuana use
*Wright & Perry (2006)	156	13–21	18.9	—	100%	Convenience	In-person interviews; quantitative	3 measures for past 30 days: (a) number of drugs used, (b) number of days used marijuana, (c) number of days used other drugs	Higher sexual identity distress associated with lower drug use
Family support and rejection									
Needham & Austin (2010)	11,153	18–26	21.8	—	1.7% gay, lesbian; 1.7% bisexual	Convenience sampling from a nationally representative school sample across the United States	Computer-assisted survey; quantitative	Marijuana and other drug use in past 30 days (other drugs listed out separately), dichotomous (yes or no)	Greater parental support associated with less drug use
Ryan, Huebner, Diaz, & Sanchez (2009)	245	21–25	22.82	—	100%	Convenience	Paper surveys; quantitative	Any illicit drug use in the past 6 months; any substance-use-related problems in the past 5 years (defined in four ways: problems with the law; loss of employment; loss of consciousness; and conflicts with family, lovers, or friends)	LGB young adults who reported rejection in adolescence were 3.4 times more likely to use illegal drugs.

Ryan, Russell, Huebner, Diaz, & Sanchez (2010)	245	21–25	Not reported	Not reported	100%	Convenience	Computer-assisted and paper surveys; quantitative	Four types of problems resulting from drug/alcohol use in past 5 years	Low levels of family acceptance were related to higher levels of substance abuse
*Padilla, Crisp, & Rew (2010)	1906	12–17	16	—	100% LGB (54.56% ay, 10.81% lesbian, 34.63% bisexual)	National convenience sample	Online surveys; quantitative	Dichotomous variable: use of marijuana, cocaine, ecstasy, or crystal meth in past 30 days	Higher likelihood of substance use among youth who experienced family rejection
Willoughby, Doty, & Malik (2010)	81	14–25	19.70	1.76	100% (54.56% gay, 10.81% lesbian, 34.63% bisexual)	Convenience	Paper questionnaire; quantitative	Personal Experience Screening Questionnaire (18 items): severity of drug use, frequency of use, problems resulting	Higher family rejection was related to increased substance use problem severity.
Elze (1999)	184	13–18	16.6	1.1	100%	Convenience	Self-administered questionnaires; quantitative	5 ordinal items from the Youth Risk Behavior Survey (YSRB); frequency of lifetime and past use of specific drugs	Negative family attitudes related to higher substance use when peer network is poor
*Espelage, Aragon, Birkett, & Koenig (2008)	13,921	High school	15.8	—	7.65% LGB, 6.69% questioning	Purposive (all students from 18 high schools in a single county)	Paper survey; quantitative	Hard drug and marijuana use	Family support moderates the relationship between homophobic teasing and drug use.
Social support									
Birkett, Espelage, & Koenig (2009)	7,367	12–14	Not reported	Not reported	13.8% of males and 9.5 % males identified as LGB	Convenience	Anonymous paper surveys; quantitative	Marijuana use frequency past 12 months	Positive perceptions of school climate associated with lower levels of marijuana use; higher rates of homophobic teasing related to higher marijuana use
Safren (1998)	104	16–21	Total sample, 18.2; LGB sample, 18.4	Total sample, 1.6; LGB sample, 1.6		Convenience	Anonymous questionnaires; quantitative	Personal Experience Screening Questionnaire (18 items): severity of drug use, frequency of use, problems resulting	Social support and coping associated with substance use by LGB sample

(*Continued*)

TABLE 1 (Continued)

Stressors and author	Sample characteristics: N	Age range	M age	SD	% LGB	Sample strategy	Data collection strategy	Substance use measure	Key findings: IV–DV relationship
Jurgensen (2013)	377	15–19	16.69	1.18	100%	Convenience	Face-to-face structured interviews and surveys; quantitative	How often in the past year for 12 different substances	Peer support was unrelated to substance use; school support was unrelated to substance use.
Boyle (2009)	30	18–25	—	—	50%	Convenience	In-person interview; qualitative	Qualitative discussion of use	Youth report substance use to fit in with peer groups and manage anxiety
*Rosario, Schrimshaw, & Hunter (2004)	156	14–21	18.3	1.65	66% LG; 31% B; 3% "free spirit or confused"	Convenience	In-person interviews; quantitative	Quantity of marijuana use (how many joints have when smoking) at each time (1–3)	Ongoing activity in LGB-related activities related to inconsistent use patterns
Housing instability									
Wright & Perry (2006)	156	13–21	18.9	—	100%	Convenience	In-person interviews; quantitative	Three measures for past 30 days: (a) number of drugs used, (b) number of days used marijuana, (c) number of days used other drugs	Leaving home associated with higher drug use
Whitbeck, Chen, Hoyt, Tyler, & Johnson (2004)	428	16–19	17.4	1.05	14.7% LGB	Convenience	Computer-assisted personal interviews; quantitative	University of Michigan Composite International Diagnostic Interview (UMCID), a revision of the CDI (assesses major depression, posttraumatic stress disorder, alcohol use, and drug use)	Drug abuse was positively associated with engaging in nonsexual street subsistence strategies among LGB adolescents.
Elze, Stiffman, & Dore (1999)	184	13–18	16.6	1.1	100%	Convenience	Self-administered Questionnaires; Quantitative	5 ordinal items from the Youth Risk Behavior Survey: frequency of lifetime and past use of drugs	Living at home associated with lower substance use

Victimization									
*Rosario, Rotheram-Borus, & Reid (1996)	136	14–19	16.8	1.4	100%	Convenience	In-person interviews; quantitative	Drug use frequency over past 3 months using a 3-point response scale	Parents discovering LGB identity, other kin discovering LGB identity, and being ridiculed by others were related to increased drug use within last 3 months.
Willoughby, Doty, & Malik (2010)	81; 10	14-25	19.70	1.76	0% (54.56% gay, 10.81% lesbian, 34.63% bisexual)	Convenience	Paper questionnaire; quantitative	Personal Experience Screening Questionnaire (18 items): severity of drug use, frequency of use, problems resulting	Being ridiculed by others was not related to increased drug use within last 3 months.
Birkett, Espelage, & Koenig (2009)	7,367	12–14	Not reported	Not reported	13.8% of males and 9.5 % males identified as LGB	Convenience	Anonymous paper surveys; quantitative	Marijuana use frequency in the past 12 months	Higher rates of homophobic teasing related to higher marijuana use.
Safren (1998)	104	16–21	Total sample, 18.2; LGB sample, 18.4	Total sample, 1.6; LGB sample, 1.6		Convenience	Anonymous questionnaires; quantitative	Personal Experience Screening Questionnaire (18 items): severity of drug use, frequency of use, problems resulting	Stress experiences related to LGB identification not associated with increased substance use among the LGB-only sample.
Jurgensen (2013)	377	15–19	16.69	1.18	100%	Convenience	Face-to-face structured interviews and questionnaires; quantitative	How often in the past year for 12 substances	Peer support unrelated to substance use; school support unrelated to substance use; victimization unrelated to substance use.
Bontempo & D'Augelli (2002)	9188	9th –12th graders	16	—	3.4%	YRBS survey through public and private schools; purposive	Paper survey; quantitative	Past month drug use; additional question of lifetime use of other street drugs	LGB youth who reported high levels of victimization at school had higher levels of substance use, and low levels of victimization were related to substance use similar to heterosexual peers

(*Continued*)

TABLE 1 (Continued)

Stressors and author	Sample characteristics: N	Age range	M age	SD	% LGB	Sample strategy	Data collection strategy	Substance use measure	Key findings: IV–DV relationship
Thoma (2012)	276	14–19	17.45	1.36	100%	Convenience	Computer-assisted questionnaire; quantitative	Marijuana use in past month (No use, 1–6 days, 7–25 days, 26 or more days)	Racist discrimination associated with increased substance use, antigay discrimination was not. There was significant interaction between these two predictors where antigay discrimination was a significant predictor only at low levels of racist discrimination.
Boyle (2009)	30	18–25	Not reported	Not reported	50%	Convenience	In-person interview; qualitative	Qualitative discussion of use	Substance use to fit in or manage anxiety
Espelage, Aragon, Birkett, & Koenig (2008)	13,921	High school	15.8	—	7.65% LGB, 6.69% questioning	Purposive (all students from 18 high schools in a single county)	Paper survey	Three items pertaining to marijuana use	LGB students who reported higher levels of homophobic teasing also reported more marijuana use than those who reported less homophobic teasing.
Russell, Ryan, Toomey, Diaz, & Sanchez (2011)	245	21–25	22.8	1.4	100%	Convenience sampling (retrospective to age 13–19)	Computer-assisted and paper surveys; quantitative	Problems due to substance use measured using four items: assessing problems with the law, losing job, passed out, conflicts with family within past 5 years	Past in-school sexual orientation victimization was not related to current substance use or abuse.
Questioning identity									
Poteat, Aragon, Espelage, & Koenig (2009)	14,439	14–19	15.86	1.22	7.4% LGB, 6.5% questioning	Convenience	Paper survey; quantitative	10-item drug use scale assessed substance use over past 12 months using a 5-point scale from 0 (*not at all*) to 5 (*daily*)	Questioning youth used more substances than LGB

Note. IV = independent variable; DV = dependent variable; LGB = lesbian, gay, or bisexual; CDI = Children's Depression Inventory.
*Indicates multiple reports from the same study.

of individuals disclosed to that predicted drug use, but it was the negative reactions by individuals, including family rejection, that predicted drug use (Rosario et al., 2009; Ryan et al., 2009). There were also meaningful differences between those who came out on their own terms versus those whose sexual identity was discovered. Specifically, LGB adolescents whose family members discovered or outed their sexual identity were more likely to engage in drug use than LGB adolescents who disclosed to their parents or other family members (Rosario et al., 1996). However, there is not a consensus on this matter, as exemplified by Wright and Perry (2006), who found that LGB youth with greater sexual identity distress reported lower rates of drug use than their peers.

Family Support and Rejection

Seven reports explored the influence of family on drug use among LGB adolescents. Espelage, Aragon, Birkett, and Koenig (2008) found that parent support moderated the relationship between homophobic teasing and marijuana use among a large school-based sample of LGB teens. Elze, Stiffman, and Dore (1999), Ryan, Russell, Huebner, Diaz, and Sanchez (2010), and Willoughby et al. (2010) found that family rejection was directly related to higher drug use. Similarly, Ryan and colleagues (2009) found that LGB youth who experienced high rates of family rejection during adolescence were 3.4 times as likely to use illicit substances compared to those who experienced no to low levels of family rejection. Moreover, increased positive support from family (Needham & Austin, 2010) and specifically a mother (Padilla et al., 2010) during the "coming out process" was related to lower rates of drug use among LGB adolescents.

Social Support

Five reports examined social support as offered through friends, peers, teachers, and, more broadly, the supportive school climate and its relationship to adolescents' drug use. Espelage and colleagues (2008) and Birkett, Espelage, and Koenig (2009) found that, similar to parental support, a supportive school environment buffers against drug use for LGB adolescents. However, the relationship between social support from peers and drug use is unclear. In a qualitative study by Boyle (2009), participants reported that LGB adolescents who reported higher rates of drug use were using as a means for fitting in with peers. Wright and Perry (2006) found that having more LGB people in youth's support networks was associated with more frequent drug use, although the effect size of this relationship was small. This same study found no significant relationship between social support of LGB people on participants' patterns of use, similar to findings from two additional studies (Jurgensen, 2013; Safren, 1998). Whereas Padilla et al. (2010) found that involvement with LGB social support such as the school-based Gay

Straight Alliance (GSA), had no effect on drug use for LGB youth, Rosario, Schrimshaw, and Hunter (2004) found that youth who were involved in LGB-related activities reported inconsistent use patterns. Finally, Willoughby and colleagues (2010) also found that being ridiculed by peers was not related to drug use among participants.

Housing Instability

Three reports indicated a positive relationship between homelessness (Elze et al., 1999; Whitbeck, Chen, Hoyt, Tyler, & Johnson, 2004) or running away from home (Wright & Perry, 2006) and drug use for LGB adolescents. Wright and Perry (2006) found that running away from home was a predictor of drug use in their sample of LGB adolescents, and Whitbeck et al. (2004) found that engagement in subsistence strategies predicted higher drug use by LGB homeless youth. In a related study, Elze et al. (1999) found that living at home was associated with lower drug use by LGB adolescents.

LGB-Related Victimization

Ten studies in this analysis explored the relationship between LGB-related victimization and drug use. Previous research has been mixed in correlating victimization to increased drug use. Bontempo and D'Augelli (2002) found that high levels of victimization were correlated with higher levels of drug use. Additionally, LGB youth who reported high victimization reported a significantly higher degree of drug use than LGB youth who reported low levels of victimization (Bontempo & D'Augelli, 2002). This same report also found that LGB youth who reported lower levels of victimization had similar rates of drug use compared to the heterosexual group. Thoma (2012) and Jurgensen (2013), on the other hand, found that antigay discrimination was not associated with drug use.

Victimization has also been explored in combination with other key variables. For example, Espelage and colleagues (2008) found that high levels of homophobic teasing were correlated with high levels of marijuana use, particularly when combined with low levels of parental support. Similarly, LGB youth who were exposed to higher levels of homophobic teasing reported more marijuana use than LGB youth who reported lower levels of homophobic teasing (Birkett et al., 2009). For homeless youth, drug use was associated with nearly twice the rate of victimization (Whitbeck et al., 2004). Victimization was also associated with the development of a negative LGB identity, internalized stigma, and subsequent drug use behaviors (Willoughby et al., 2010). Another study found that LGB youth who experienced a positive school climate reported lower levels of marijuana use than LGB youth who did not experience a positive school climate (Birkett et al., 2009). However, a more recent study found that higher levels of victimization were related to susceptibility to mental health problems, previous suicide attempt, and engagement in HIV and sexually transmitted infection (STI) risk behaviors but not drug use (Russell et al., 2011). Three additional studies (Jurgensen, 2013; Safren, 1998; Willoughby et al., 2010) also found no relationship between victimization and drug use.

Questioning Identity

Poteat, Aragon, Espelage, and Koenig (2009) found that identifying as "questioning" was associated with higher rates of drug use than identifying as LGB. Although we do not extend that this identity is in and of itself a risk factor, we included it in our review as it highlights a particular need for future research (described later).

DISCUSSION

Our study supports the use of minority stress theory in understanding trauma and drug use among LGB adolescents, with some important nuance. Psychological stress, including the experience of internalized homophobia, was often discussed, yet far from universally agreed on. Although a number of reports found a relationship between psychological stress and drug use, one study found the relationship to be significant for females only (Rotheram-Borus, Rosario, Van Rossem, Reid, & Gillis, 1995). Further, whereas Wright and Perry (2006) found that sexual identity distress was negatively associated with drug use, two other reports (Rosario et al., 2004, 2009) found no relationship at all. These reports indicate that psychological distress might operate differently across gender and sexual orientation, an important area for future research. Further, as sexual identity distress tends to lessen as an individual becomes more comfortable in his or her sexual identity (Meyer, 2003), measuring this construct should include an understanding of an individual's context regarding his or her personal disclosure process within his or her social network and larger community.

The presence of a supportive network is commonly cited as a buffer against the impact of trauma (Cohen, Underwood, & Gottlieb, 2000), and both family and social support were considered in our review. Lending to the importance of "disclosure-related trauma" in understanding drug use, family support during the coming out process appeared to buffer against drug use (Espelage et al., 2008; Padilla et al., 2010; Ryan et al., 2010). Similarly, LGB youth who experienced family rejection were 3.4 times as likely to use illicit substances (Ryan et al., 2010). However, no studies used valid measures of family support or rejection within the context of the LGB experience, and further research is needed to understand this dynamic relationship (Bouris et al., 2011).

Social support by peers was also discussed; however, having supportive peers did not necessarily buffer against drug use when youth report concurrent negative disclosure reactions (Rosario et al., 2009). Further, although being around youth who are similar might impact an individual's perception of self, youth who participate in social milieu such as GSAs might actually report increases in use (Boyle, 2009; Rosario et al., 2004; Safren, 1998). We again ally this uptake in drug use with disclosure-related victimization commonly experienced by youth who openly identified as LGB in high school (Garofalo et al., 1998). Additionally, peer networks could function as social environments where drug use is accepted and common. Therefore, supportive peer networks might not function to decrease drug use, but could provide other psychosocial benefits.

These findings have important implications for practitioners: When a youth becomes identified with the LGB community, is he or she at greater risk for drug use? Studies have found that earlier age of disclosure or difficulty in hiding sexual orientation was related to increased LGB adolescents' susceptibility for substance abuse (Pilkington & D'Augelli, 1995). However, exposure to traumatic minority stress experiences after disclosure likely increases, perhaps lending to this outcome. At the same time, identification with a community that has experienced significant marginalization over time can also increase an individual's susceptibility to drug use patterns (McNaughton, 2008). Some research on the impact of historical trauma and community grief (Brave Heart, Chase, Elkins, & Altschul, 2011) might elucidate this dynamic relationship, and suggest a need for more structural interventions. Additionally, one study in our review (Birkett et al., 2009) found that a positive school climate and low levels of victimization (as opposed to high levels) served as buffers against drug use among LGB adolescents. Further research underscoring both the risks associated with marginalization and the buffers that mitigate these risks is warranted.

Although we did not consider sexual orientation as a risk factor directly, we opted to leave in one study that found that youth who identified as questioning were at higher risk for drug use (Poteat et al., 2009). This study highlights the need for more research on subgroup differences on minority stress experiences among sexual minority youth. Similarly, although bisexual youth were included in many of the studies in our analysis, more research is needed to understand differences between distinct groups of lesbian, bisexual, and gay youth. For instance, Marshal et al. (2009) found heterogeneity in a meta-analysis of sexual orientation and drug use patterns, with bisexual youth and females using substances significantly more than other sexual minority groups.

Study Limitations

Limitations of this review serve to highlight limitations in the available literature. Of particular concern is the lack of standardization concerning which ages constitute an "adolescent" or "youth," with studies ranging in populations of 13 to 25. Initially, the authors wished to restrict this review to only those studies that described an adolescent population between 13 and 18 years of age. This limited scope would have drastically reduced the total available reports, making the current synthesis impossible. Other authors have also written about this concern (Elze, 2007) and future research should explore the effect of employing stricter guidelines. In short, the experience of a 25-year-old participant likely does not represent the experiences of a 15-year-old. As we expanded to studies with participants retrospectively reporting on their adolescence, recall bias might be an issue particularly as it relates to memory of traumatic experiences (Williams, 1994). Additionally, although some of the included studies described their samples as including transgender youth, we believed that this review would have been misleading if it referred broadly to the sample of participants as LGBT. The needs of transgender adolescents are often quite different from their sexual orientation minority peers and this review of sexual minority youth could not effectively address the unique experience of transgender youth (Kosciw, Greytak, Bartkiewicz, Boesen, & Palmer, 2012).

Although research indicates we are not yet "post-gay" (Russell, Clarke, & Clary, 2009), some sexual minority adolescents might also not ascribe to a specific LGB identity label or might feel unsafe disclosing their sexual identity. Therefore, many of the analyses presented here could have systematically missed a group of young people who do not identify within rigid sexual identity labels but still face similar challenges as those who do identify as LGB.

The majority of studies included in this systematic review were cross-sectional and lacked longitudinal findings that make it impossible to examine causal relationships. Our generalizability is also affected in several ways. First, very few of the included reports used nationally representative samples or were qualitative. Further, these reports span over two decades (from 1990–2013) and a number of human rights advances have been made (e.g., the repeal of Don't Ask, Don't Tell in the military) that might impact broader perception and experience of LGB adolescents in the present day. A number of included reports (e.g., Rosario et al., 1997; Rosario et al., 2004, 2008; Rosario, Schrimshaw, Hunter, & Gwadz, 2002) came from the same initial study, which might introduce bias into our reporting. However, as these studies reported on different stress factors and their relationship to drug use, we believed it best to list them separately within the table and our report. As in any review, we were only able to summarize information that authors chose to report; it is possible that previous studies did investigate the relationship between minority stressors and drug use but did not report them for lack of significant findings. We tried to guard against this by including unpublished literature. Included studies rarely discussed racial and ethnic differences across participants, with few exceptions (e.g., Rosario et al., 2004; Ryan et al., 2009). There continues to be a dearth of research on the relationship between the unique experiences of racially and ethnically diverse LGB adolescents and drug use.

Overwhelmingly, it seems that many forms of minority stress appear to cooccur within individuals. That is, LGB adolescents who are homeless often experience family rejection, victimization related to their sexual orientation, and other stressors. Thus, more nuanced and multifactored research on minority stress is needed; exploring the effects of a single stressor might not be as useful as the examination of simultaneous effects of many minority stressors as they occur in young peoples' experiences. As we look toward developing interventions that can prevent, intervene on, and treat drug use behaviors among LGB adolescents, we should endeavor to address these numerous minority stress factors simultaneously. A more holistic approach to understanding both the etiology of behavioral health disparities among LGB youth, as well as the development of coping and behavioral change strategies, will likely find more positive benefit.

Implications of Findings

It is clear that the various stress factors related to drug use among LGB adolescents are overlapping and complicated. Only one category, family support, seemed to be clearly associated with drug use patterns across studies. This finding emphasized the need for family-based interventions such as those supported by the Family Acceptance Project (Ryan et al., 2010). Other studies of minority stress domains presented more heterogeneous findings. Based on our analysis, we believe this is influenced by a number of factors. First, researchers must work to further operationalize measures of minority stress for LGB adolescents. For example, although some studies did differentiate between general and gay-related victimization, considering these measures of victimization simultaneously might be clouding our understanding of their differences, making it difficult to assess the degree to which victimization is targeting LGB identity alone or if other stigmatized aspects of a person or population are being targeted. This suggests a need for the development of well-validated measures of minority stress for LGB adolescents so that future researchers can more accurately test hypotheses of minority stress in relations to their use of substances.

REFERENCES

Alessi, E. J., Meyer, I. H., & Martin, J. I. (2013). PTSD and sexual orientation: An examination of criterion A1 and non-criterion A1 events. *Psychological Trauma: Theory, Research, Practice, and Policy*, *5*, 149–157. doi:10.1037/a0026642

Almeida, J., Johnson, R. M., Corliss, H. L., Molnar, B. E., & Azreal, D. (2009). Emotional distress among LGBT youth: The influence of perceived discrimination based on sexual orientation. *Journal of Youth and Adolescence, 38*, 1001–1014. doi:10.1007/10964-009-9408-x

Alvy, L. M., Hughes, T. L., Kristjanson, A. F., & Wilsnack, S. C. (2013). Sexual identity group differences in child abuse and neglect. *Journal of Interpersonal Violence*, 1–24. doi:10.1177/0886260512471081

Bailey, N. J., & Phariss, T. (1996). Breaking through the wall of silence: Gay, lesbian, and bisexual issues for middle level educators. *Middle School Journal, 27*, 38–46.

Balsam, K. F., Rothblum, E. D., & Beauchaine, T. P. (2005). Victimization over the life span: A comparison of lesbian, gay, bisexual, and heterosexual siblings. *Journal of Consulting and Clinical Psychology, 73*, 477–487. doi:10.1037/0022-006X.73.3.477

Birkett, M., Espelage, D. L., & Koenig, B. (2009). LGB and questioning students in schools: The moderating effects of homophobic bullying and school climate on negative outcomes. *Journal of Youth and Adolescence, 38*, 989–1000. doi:10.1007/s10964-008-9389-1

Bontempo, D. E., & D'Augelli, A. R. (2002). Effects of at-school victimization and sexual orientation on lesbian, gay, or bisexual youths' health risk behavior. *Journal of Adolescent Health, 30*, 364–374. doi:10.1016/S1054-139X(01)00415-3

Bouris, A., Guilamo-Ramos, V., Jaccard, J., Ballan, M., Lesesne, C. A., & Gonzalez, B. (2011). Early adolescent romantic relationships and maternal approval among inner city Latino families. *AIDS and Behavior, 16*, 1570–1583. doi:10.1007/s10461-011-0034-8

Boyle, T. J. (2009). *The experiences of homeless lesbian, gay, bisexual, and transgender youth and the meanings attached to these experiences* (Doctoral dissertation). Retrieved from Proquest. (UMI 3401429)

Brave Heart, M. Y. H., Chase, J., Elkins, J., & Altschul, D. B. (2011). Historical trauma among indigenous peoples of the Americas: Concepts, research, and clinical considerations. *Journal of Psychoactive Drugs, 43*, 282–290. doi:10.1080/02791072.2011.628913

Cervantes, R. C., & Goldbach, J. T. (2012). Adapting evidence-based prevention approaches for Latino adolescents: The Familia Adelante Program–Revised Adaptación de Programas de Prevención Basados en la Evidencia para Adolescentes Hispanos: El Programa Familia Adelante–Revisado. *Psychosocial Intervention, 21*, 281–290.

Clatts, M. C., Goldsamt, L., Huso, Y., & Gwadz, M. V. (2005). Homelessness and drug abuse among young men who have sex with men in New York City: A preliminary epidemiological trajectory. *Journal of Adolescence, 28*, 201–214. doi:10.1016/j.adolescence.2005.02.003

Cohen, S., Underwood, L. G., & Gottlieb, B. (Eds.). (2000). *Social support measurement and intervention: A guide for health and social scientists*. New York, NY: Oxford University Press.

Corliss, H. L., Rosario, M., Wypij, D., Wylie, S. A., Frazier, A. L., & Austin, S. B. (2010). Sexual orientation and drug use in a longitudinal cohort study of U.S. adolescents. *Addictive Behaviors, 35*, 517–521. doi:10.1016/j.addbeh.2009.12.019

D'Augelli, A. R., & Grossman, A. H. (2001). Disclosure of sexual orientation, victimization, and mental health among lesbian, gay, and bisexual older adults. *Journal of Interpersonal Violence, 16*, 1008–1027. doi:10.1177/088626001016010003

Elze, D. E. (2007). Research with sexual minority youth. *Journal of Gay and Lesbian Social Services, 18*, 73–99. doi:10.1300/J041v18n02_05

Elze, D. E., Stiffman, A. R., & Dore, P. (1999). The association between types of violence exposure and youths' mental health problems. *International Journal of Adolescent Medicine and Health, 11*, 221–256. doi:10.1515/IJAMH.1999.11.3-4.221

Espelage, D. L., Aragon, S. R., Birkett, M., & Koenig, B. W. (2008). Homophobic teasing, psychological outcomes, and sexual orientation among high school students: What influence do parents and schools have? *School Psychology Review, 37*, 202–216.

Follette, V. M., Polusny, M. A., Bechtle, A. E., & Naugle, A. E. (1996). Cumulative trauma: The impact of child sexual abuse, adult sexual assault, and spouse abuse. *Journal of Traumatic Stress, 9*, 25–35. doi:10.1007/BF02116831

Gaddis, L. K. (2011). *Growing up lesbian in the rural deep south: "I only knew I was different"* (Doctoral dissertation). Retrieved from ProQuest. (UMI 3450292)

Garofalo, R., Wolf, R. C., Kessel, S., Palfrey, J., & DuRant, R. H. (1998). The association between health risk behaviors and sexual orientation among a school-based sample of adolescents. *Pediatrics, 101*, 895–902. doi:10.1542/peds.101.5.895

Gilmore, T. C. (1996). *Stress, coping, and adjustment among gay, lesbian, and bisexual youth* (Doctoral dissertation). Retrieved from ProQuest. (UMI 9625607)

Goldbach, J. T., & Holleran Steiker, L. K. (2011). An examination of cultural adaptations performed by LGBT-identified youths to a culturally grounded, evidence-based substance abuse intervention. *Journal of Gay & Lesbian Social Services, 23*, 188–203. doi:10.1080/10538720.2011.560135

Goldbach, J. T., Tanner-Smith, E. E., Bagwell, M., & Dunlap, S. (2014). Minority stress and drug use in sexual minority adolescents: A meta-analysis. *Prevention Science, 15*, 350–363. doi:10.1007/s11121-013-0393-7

Goodman, L. A., Corcoran, C., Turner, K., Yuan, N., & Green, B. L. (1998). Assessing traumatic event exposure: General issues and preliminary findings for the Stressful Life Events Screening Questionnaire. *Journal of Traumatic Stress, 11*, 521–542. doi:10.1023/A:1024456713321

Grossman, A. H., Haney, A. P., Edwards, P., Alessi, E. J., Ardon, M., & Howell, T. J. (2009). Lesbian, gay, bisexual and transgender youth talk about experiencing and coping with school violence: A qualitative study. *Journal of LGBT Youth, 6*, 24–46. doi:10.1080/19361650802379748

Haas, A. P., Eliason, M., Mays, V. M., Mathy, R. M., Cochran, S. D., D'Augelli, A. R., . . . Clayton, P. J. (2010). Suicide and suicide risk in lesbian, gay, bisexual, and transgender populations: Review and recommendations. *Journal of Homosexuality, 58*, 10–51. doi:10.1080/00918369.2011.534038

Hatzenbuehler, M. L., Pachankis, J. E., & Wolff, J. (2012). Religious climate and health risk behaviors in sexual minority youths: A population-based study. *Journal Information, 102*, 657–663. doi:10.2105/AJPH.2011.300517

Herek, G. M. (2009). Hate crimes and stigma-related experiences among sexual minority adults in the United States: Prevalence estimates from a national probability sample. *Journal of Interpersonal Violence, 24*, 54–74. doi:10.1177/0886260508316477

Hughes, T. L., & Eliason, M. (2002). Coming-out process related to drug use among gay, lesbian and bisexual teens. *The Brown University Digest of Addiction Theory & Application*, *24*, 3–4.

Jurgensen, E. K. (2013). *Examining social support as a factor promoting resiliency against negative outcomes among sexual minority youth* (Doctoral dissertation). Retrieved from ProQuest. (UMI 3564817)

Kosciw, J. G., Greytak, E. A., Bartkiewicz, M. J., Boesen, M. J., & Palmer, N. A. (2012). *The 2011 National School Climate Survey: The experiences of lesbian, gay, bisexual and transgender youth in our nation's schools*. New York, NY: GLSEN.

Kosciw, J. G., Palmer, N. A., Kull, R. M., & Greytak, E. A. (2013). The effect of negative school climate on academic outcomes for LGBT youth and the role of in-school supports. *Journal of School Violence*, *12*, 45–63. doi:10.1080/15388220.2012.732546

Marshal, M. P., Friedman, M. S., Stall, R., King, K. M., Miles, J., Gold, M. A., & Morse, J. Q. (2008). Sexual orientation and adolescent drug use: A meta-analysis and methodological review. *Addiction*, *103*, 546–556. doi:10.1111/j.1360-0443.2008.02149.x

Marshal, M. P., Friedman, M. S., Stall, R., & Thompson, A. L. (2009). Individual trajectories of drug use in lesbian, gay and bisexual youth and heterosexual youth. *Addiction*, *104*, 974–981. doi:10.1111/j.1360-0443.2009.02531.x

McNaughton, C. C. (2008). Transitions through homelessness, drug use, and the effect of material marginalization and psychological trauma. *Drugs: Education, Prevention, and Policy*, *15*, 177–188. doi:10.1080/09687630701377587

Meyer, I. H. (2003). Prejudice, social stress, and mental health in lesbian, gay, and bisexual populations: Conceptual issues and research evidence. *Psychological Bulletin*, *129*, 674–697. doi:10.1037/0033-2909.129.5.674

Moher, D., Liberati, A., Tetzlaff, J., Altman, D. G., & The PRISMA Group. (2009). Preferred reporting items for systematic reviews and meta-analyses: The PRISMA statement. *PLoS Med*, *6*(6), e1000097. doi:10.1371/journal.pmed1000097

Moon, M. W., Fornili, K., & O'Briant, A. L. (2007). Risk comparison among youth who report sex with same-sex versus both-sex partners. *Youth & Society*, *38*, 267–284. doi:10.1177/0044118X06287689

National Institute on Drug Abuse. *Comorbidity: Addiction and other mental health illnesses* (2008).

Needham, B. L., & Austin, E. L. (2010). Sexual orientation, parent support, and health during the transition into adulthood. *Journal of Youth and Adolescence*, *39*, 1189–1198. doi:10.1007/s10964-010-9533-6

Padilla, Y. C., Crisp, C., & Rew, D. L. (2010). Parental acceptance and illegal drug use among gay, lesbian, and bisexual adolescents: Results from a national survey. *Social Work*, *55*, 265–275. doi:10.1093/sw/55.3.26

Pilkington, N. W., & D'Augelli, A. R. (1995). Victimization of lesbian, gay, and bisexual youth in community settings. *Journal of Community Psychology*, *23*, 34–56. doi:10.1002/1520-6629

Poteat, V. P., Aragon, S. R., Espelage, D. L., & Koenig, B. W. (2009). Psychosocial concerns of sexual minority youth: Complexity and caution in-group differences. *Journal of Consulting and Clinical Psychology*, *77*, 196–201. doi:10.1037/a0014158

Remafedi, G. (1987). Adolescent homosexuality: Psychological and medical implications. *Pediatrics*, *79*, 331–337.

Roberts, A. L., Austin, S. B., Corliss, H. L., Vandermorris, A. K., & Koenen, K. C. (2010). Pervasive trauma exposure among US sexual orientation minority adults and risk of posttraumatic stress disorder. *American Journal of Public Health*, *100*, 2433–2441.

Rosario, M., Hunter, J., & Gwadz, M. (1997). Exploration of drug use among lesbian, gay, and bisexual youth: Prevalence and correlates. *Journal of Adolescent Research*, *12*, 454–476. doi:10.1177/0743554897124003

Rosario, M., Rotheram-Borus, M., & Reid, H. (1996). Gay-related stress and its correlates among gay and bisexual male adolescents of predominantly black and Hispanic background. *Journal of Community Psychology*, *24*, 136–159. doi:10.1002/(SICI)1520-6629(199604)24:2<136::AID-JCOP5>3.0.CO;2-X

Rosario, M., Schrimshaw, E. W., & Hunter, J. (2004). Predictors of drug use over time among gay, lesbian, and bisexual youths: An examination of three hypotheses. *Addictive Behaviors*, *29*, 1623–1631. doi:10.1016/j.addbeh.2004.02.032

Rosario, M., Schrimshaw, E., & Hunter, J. (2008). Butch/Femme differences in drug use and abuse among young lesbian and bisexual women: Examination and potential explanations. *Drug Use & Misuse*, *43*, 1002–1015. doi:10.1080/10826080801914402

Rosario, M., Schrimshaw, E., & Hunter, J. (2009). Disclosure of sexual orientation and subsequent drug use and abuse among lesbian, gay, and bisexual youths: Critical role of disclosure reactions. *Psychology of Addictive Behavior*, *23*, 175–184. doi:10.1037/a0014284

Rosario, M., Schrimshaw, E. W., Hunter, J., & Gwadz, M. (2002). Gay-related stress and emotional distress among gay, lesbian and bisexual youths: A longitudinal examination. *Journal of Consulting and Clinical Psychology*, *70*, 967–975. doi:10.1037/0022-006X.70.4.967

Rotheram-Borus, M. J., Rosario, M., Van Rossem, R., Reid, H., & Gillis, R. (1995). Prevalence, course, and predictors of multiple problem behaviors among gay and bisexual male adolescents. *Developmental Psychology*, *31*, 75–85. doi:10.1037/0012-1649.31.1.75

Rowell, K., & Thomely, R. (2013). *Recovering emotionally from disaster*. Retrieved from http://www.apa.org/helpcenter/recovering-disasters.aspx.

Russell, S. T., Clarke, T. J., & Clary, J. (2009). Are teens "post-gay"? Contemporary adolescents' sexual identity labels. *Journal of Youth and Adolescence*, *38*, 884–890. doi:10.1007/s10964-008-9388-2

Russell, S. T., Driscoll, A. K., & Truong, N. (2002). Adolescent same-sex romantic attractions and relationships: Implications for drug use and abuse. *American Journal of Public Health*, *922*, 198–202.

Russell, S. T., Ryan, C., Toomey, R. B., Diaz, R. M., & Sanchez, J. (2011). Lesbian, gay, bisexual, and transgender adolescent school victimization: Implications for young adult health and adjustment. *Journal of School Health*, *81*, 223–230. doi:10.1111/j.1746-1561.2011.00583.x

Ryan, C., Huebner, D., Diaz, R. M., & Sanchez, J. (2009). Family rejection as a predictor of negative health outcomes in white and Latino lesbian, gay, and bisexual young adults. *Pediatrics*, *123*, 346–352. doi:10.1542/peds.2007-3524

Ryan, C., Russell, S. T., Huebner, D., Diaz, R., & Sanchez, J. (2010). Family acceptance in adolescence and the health of LGBT young adults. *Journal of Child and Adolescent Psychiatric Nursing, 23*, 205–213. doi:10.1111/j.1744-6171.2010.00246.x

Safren, S. A. (1998). *Depression, drug use, and suicidality in sexual minority adolescents* (Doctoral dissertation). Retrieved from ProQuest. (UMI 9806202)

Savin-Williams, R. C., & Ream, G. L. (2003). Suicide attempts among sexual-minority male youth. *Journal of Clinical Child and Adolescent Psychology, 32*, 509–522. doi:10.1207/S15374424JCCP3204_3

Thoma, B. C. (2012). *Health consequences of racist and anti-gay discrimination for multiple minority adolescents* (Doctoral dissertation). Retrieved from ProQuest. (UMI 1516290)

Toomey, R. B., Ryan, C., Diaz, R. M., & Russell, S. T. (2011). High school gay–straight alliances (GSAs) and young adult well-being: An examination of GSA presence, participation, and perceived effectiveness. *Applied Developmental Science, 15*, 175–185. doi:10.1080/10888691.2011.607378

U.S. Department of Health and Human Services, Healthy People 2020. (2011). *Lesbian, gay, bisexual, and transgender health*. Retrieved from http://www.healthypeople.gov/2020/topicsobjectives2020/overview.aspx?topicid=25

U.S. Department of Health and Human Services, Substance Abuse and Mental Health Services Administration. (2011). *A provider's introduction to substance abuse treatment for lesbian, gay, bisexual and transgender individuals*. Retrieved from http://store.samhsa.gov/product/A-Provider-s-Introduction-to-Substance-Abuse-Treatment-for-Lesbian-Gay-Bisexual-and-Transgender-Individuals/SMA 12-4104

Whitbeck, L., Chen, X., Hoyt, D., Tyler, K., & Johnson, K. (2004). Mental disorder, subsistence strategies, and victimization among gay, lesbian, and bisexual homeless and runaway adolescents. *The Journal of Sex Research, 41*, 329–342. doi:10.1080/00224490409552240

White, H. D. (1994). Scientific communication and literature retrieval. In H. Cooper & L. V. Hedges (Eds.), *The handbook of research synthesis* (pp. 41–56). New York, NY: Russell Sage Foundation.

Williams, M. L. (1994). Recall of childhood trauma: A prospective study of women's memories of child sexual abuse. *Journal of Consulting and Clinical Psychology, 62*, 1167–1176. doi:10.1037/0022-006X.62.6.1167

Willoughby, B., Doty, N., & Malik, N. (2010). Victimization, family rejection, and outcomes of gay, lesbian, and bisexual young people: The role of negative GLB identity. *Journal of GLBT Family Studies, 6*, 403–424. doi:10.1080/1550428X.2010.511085

Wright, E. R., & Perry, B. L. (2006). Sexual identity distress, social support and the health of gay, lesbian and bisexual youth. *Journal of Homosexuality, 51*, 81–110. doi:10.1300/J082v51n01_05

Young, R. M., & Meyer, I. H. (2005). The trouble with "MSM" and "WSW": Erasure of the sexual-minority person in public health discourse. *American Journal of Public Health, 95*, 1144–1149. doi:10.2105/AJPH.2004.046714

Factors Related to the Delivery of Trauma Services in Outpatient Treatment Programs

JOSEPH J. SHIELDS, PHD
Professor, National Catholic School of Social Service, The Catholic University of America, Washington, DC, USA

PETER J. DELANY, PHD
Director, Center for Behavioral Health Statistics and Quality, Substance Abuse and Mental Health Services Administration, Rockville, Maryland, USA

KELLEY E. SMITH, PHD
Project Director, Center for Behavioral Health Statistics and Quality, Substance Abuse and Mental Health Services Administration, Rockville, Maryland, USA

In recent years there has been growing recognition of the role of trauma in substance abuse treatment; however, only 20% of outpatient treatment programs report offering trauma services. We conducted a secondary analysis of the 2012 National Survey of Substance Abuse Treatment Services (N-SSATS) and explore how demographic, population served, and organization variables distinguish those programs that offer trauma services from those that do not. In this article, we present the findings, which revealed that organizational structure, process, and population served variables were the most important predictors of trauma services. Implications for social work practice in the addictions are discussed.

In recent years there has been an increased recognition of the impact of trauma on substance use disorders and the need to include trauma services for those enrolled in substance abuse treatment programs (Substance

Abuse and Mental Health Services Administration [SAMHSA], 2014). Data from both epidemiological public health surveys and studies of clients and treatment programs document a relationship between exposure to traumatic events and increases in substance use suggesting that such exposure might put individuals at increased risk for the development of substance use disorders (Davidson, Hughes, Blazer, & George, 1991; Farley, Golding, Young, Mulligan, & Minkoff, 2004; Fetzner, McMillan, Sareen, & Asmundson, 2011; Kessler, Sonnega, Bromet, Hughes, & Nelson, 1995). National population estimates suggest that the majority of individuals seeking substance abuse treatment receive services in outpatient settings (SAMHSA, 2013b). Yet, results from the National Survey of Substance Abuse Treatment Services (N-SSATS), the national survey of all known substance abuse treatment facilities, reveal that only approximately 20% of outpatient treatment programs report specifically offering trauma-related services to their clients (SAMHSA, 2013a). This percentage is similar to the findings reported by Capezza and Najavits (2012), who found that 21.3% of all reporting treatment programs offered trauma services always or often.

Given this documented need, why is it that the majority of treatment providers are not explicitly incorporating trauma services into their treatment practice? Rogers's (2003) work on the diffusion of innovative technologies in organizations has served as the foundation for a growing body of research looking at the adoption of evidence-based technologies across a number of service settings. In the substance abuse treatment literature a number of studies have examined organizational factors that relate to the adoption of pharmacotherapy interventions (Abraham & Roman, 2010; Ducharme, Knudsen, Roman, & Johnson, 2007), contingency management (Bride, Abraham, & Roman, 2011), other treatment innovations (Knudsen & Roman, 2004; Simpson, 2002), and comprehensive services (Delany, Shields, & Roberts, 2009). Bride et al. (2011) noted that there are relatively few studies that focus on the adoption of psychosocial innovations in outpatient treatment settings. The purpose of this study is to address the gap in research on psychosocial interventions for trauma by examining selected demographic variables, types of populations served, and organizational variables associated with the adoption of trauma services in outpatient substance abuse treatment facilities.

LITERATURE REVIEW

Trauma Services

Innovations in the development of trauma services emerged out of a long history within the helping professions that sought to understand and address psychological trauma. Within the last two decades, the trauma-informed care paradigm has emerged to describe approaches to address trauma from an organizational and systemic perspective (SAMHSA, 2014).

From as early as 440 BC, literature demonstrates an awareness of the psychological sequelae resulting from exposure to traumatic events and evolving treatment efforts (Crocq & Crocq, 2000; Van der Kolk, 2007). The current paradigm for understanding and addressing these sequelae is captured by the 1980 inclusion of the diagnosis of posttraumatic stress disorder (PTSD) in the *Diagnostic and Statistical Manual of Mental Disorders* (3rd ed. [*DSM–III*]; American Psychiatric Association, 1980). As research has progressed, revisions to the diagnosis have been made. Over the years, researchers, health and mental health professionals, and practitioners seeking to understand trauma developed and tested numerous specific treatments for trauma. Studies have shown success with treatments such as cognitive-behavioral therapy (CBT), prolonged exposure therapy (PE), stress inoculation therapy (SIT), and eye movement desensitization and reprocessing (EMDR; SAMHSA, 2014). As these treatments emerged to alleviate the debilitating effects of trauma, researchers also were assessing the role the overall organizational structure and treatment systems play in the healing and recovery process (Harris & Fallot, 2001). For example, in their book, *Using Trauma Theory to Design Service Systems*, Harris and Fallot (2001) articulate the important role treatment systems play in preventing the retraumatization of clients.

Populations Served

The research literature indicates that members of specific cultural and ethnic racial groups have higher rates of trauma exposure. For example, Roberts, Gilman, Breslau, Breslau, and Koenen (2011) found that African American men were significantly more likely than White men to have been violently assaulted. In the same study, African American men were significantly more likely than White men to have PTSD at some point in their lives. There is also research evidence that suggests that Latinos have higher rates of PTSD than African Americans and Whites (Pole, Gone, & Kulkarni, 2008).

The research evidence indicates that men are more likely than women to experience a traumatic event (Olf, Langeland, Draijer, & Gersons, 2007). However, women are more likely than men to experience intimate partner violence and sexual assault (Pratchett, Pelcovitz, & Yehuda, 2010). There is also evidence that women exposed to trauma tend to develop prolonged PTSD (Holbrook, Hoyt, Stein, & Sieber, 2002).

Besides these ethnic, racial, and gender differences in trauma exposure, there is evidence that people with other unique characteristics or experiences have high rates of exposure to trauma. These include people with cognitive or physical disabilities (Petersilia, 2001), homeless people (Greenberg &

Rosenheck, 2010), veterans (Kimerling et al., 2010), older people (Truman, 2011), and refugees (Nickerson, Bryant, Silove, & Steel, 2011).

These findings highlight the need for substance abuse treatment providers to have a thorough understanding of the unique needs of the clients they serve. For example, programs that serve large numbers of women should be attuned to issues of intimate partner violence and sexual assault, whereas programs that serve veterans and refugees need to have an understanding of the effects of exposure to combat and war in designing treatment plans.

Organizational Variables

In response to the research to practice gap (Lamb, Greenlick, & McCarty, 1998), a significant number of addiction health services research studies have focused on factors that can help explain the resistance to the adoption of evidence-based treatment practices that most treatment facilities exhibit (Roman & Johnson, 2002). To understand how treatment programs adopt innovative practices, researchers have conducted case studies of the technology transfer in individual treatment programs (Liddle et al., 2002; Martin, Herie, Turner, & Cunningham, 1998). Studies have also focused on the characteristics of the clinical workforce (Ball et al., 2002; Forman, Bovasso, & Woody, 2001: Knudsen, Ducharme, Roman, & Link, 2005). Other researchers have focused on organizational structures and processes to understand the adoption of treatment innovations (Rosenheck, 2001; Simpson, 2002). In attempting to understand the organizational characteristics related to the adoption of naltrexone in private substance abuse treatment programs, Roman and Johnson (2002) studied factors such as ownership, size, leadership, and caseload characteristics. In a similar study on the adoption of buprenorphine in treatment programs, Knudsen, Ducharme, and Roman (2006) studied organizational factors such as ownership, size, accreditation, and staffing characteristics. In a study on the adoption of psychosocial innovations (e.g., contingency management), Bride, Abraham, and Roman (2010) studied structural factors such as ownership, size, and accreditation.

To further the understanding of organizational processes and the adoption of innovation in treatment programs Knudsen and Roman (2004) introduced the concept of *absorptive capacity,* defined as the ability of an organization to access and effectively use information. The concept has been used by organizational theorists to explain the adoption of new technologies and services in a variety of industries (Knudsen & Roman, 2004). They stated, "organizations with greater information processing and application capabilities are more likely to use innovations" (Knudsen & Roman, 2004, p. 51). They then model the relationship between absorptive capacity and the use of treatment innovations by focusing on workforce professionalism, environmental scanning, and the collection of satisfaction data. Although these are clearly important dimensions of absorptive capacity, other factors such as internal and external case review practices, as well as periodic utilization review, are important learning strategies for treatment facilities.

The research literature indicates the importance of including organizational structure and process variables, as well as variables related to client characteristics and populations served, in developing models explaining the adoption of treatment innovations for substance abuse treatment programs.

THIS STUDY

In this study we use data derived from a national survey of substance abuse treatment facilities to assess the extent to which selected demographic variables, population served variables, and organizational structure and process variables predict the extent to which treatment programs incorporate trauma-informed services into practice.

METHODS

Data Source

This study employed a secondary analysis of the 2012 N-SSATS. The N-SSATS is an annual survey conducted by SAMHSA of all known substance abuse treatment programs in the United States and its jurisdictions (SAMHSA, 2013a). The survey collects data about facility characteristics, number of clients served, types of services provided, and the availability of programs for specific populations. No information is obtained directly from clients. The surveys were sent to the facilities administrators and were completed by the administrators or their designees.

In 2012 the N-SSATS collected data from a total of 14,311 substance abuse treatment facilities. For this study, we selected only those facilities that offered substance abuse treatment services and those whose primary focus was substance abuse treatment. This eliminated programs that only provided intake or referral services, and those that provided only detoxification services. It also eliminated those programs whose primary focus was mental health services or general health care. We further pared down the sample by selecting only those programs that were either regular or intensive outpatient treatment programs. This eliminated the hospital inpatient programs, residential programs, and methadone programs. We also eliminated those programs not located in the 50 states or the District of Columbia. This process resulted in a final sample of 4,762 facilities or 33% of the original data set.

Measures

Trauma services

The questionnaire included a list of therapeutic approaches that are used in substance abuse treatment. The respondents were asked to rate each in terms how often the approach was used in their facility. For this analysis we selected the "trauma-related counseling" item and coded the responses so that *never, rarely,* or *sometimes* equaled 0 and *always or often* equaled 1.

Demographic characteristics

Two demographic characteristics were included in the analysis. Region of the country was categorized as the Northeast, Midwest, South, and West. The second variable was a measure of urbanicity. The location of each facility was rated on a 6-point scale from least urban to most urban. The rating scale was developed by the National Center on Health Statistics and is commonly used in national health surveys (Ingram & Franco, 2013).

Populations served

The questionnaire asked the respondents to report on the types of clients accepted into treatment and whether the facility offered specifically designed programs for the population. For this analysis we selected six groups that often present themselves in treatment with trauma-related issues. These groups included adolescents, people with cooccurring mental and substance use disorders, criminal justice clients, adult women, pregnant women, and veterans. Organizations that reported having programs for these groups were scored 1 and those that did not have programs were scored 0.

Organizational characteristics

The organizational variables that were included in this study were ownership, size, financing characteristics, accreditation, and absorptive capacity. Ownership was a dichotomous variable that contrasted not-for-profit facilities with for-profit facilities. Organizational size was measured by the total number of clients who received intensive or regular outpatient services during March 2012. The distribution was recoded into five quintiles. Three financing variables were included in the analysis: Did the facility use a sliding fee scale? Did the facility offer treatment at no charge to clients? Did the facility receive any government funding or grants? The responses to these three items were coded so that yes equaled 1 and no equaled 0. Two accreditation measures were included in the analysis: whether the facility was accredited by the Joint Commission on the Accreditation of Health Care

Organizations (JCAHCO), and whether the facility was accredited by the Council on Accreditation (COA).

Absorptive capacity, defined as an organization's capacity to access and effectively use information (Knudsen & Roman, 2004), was measured by the responses to whether or not the following practices were part of the standard operating procedures of the facility: (a) required continuing education for staff, (b) conducted periodic drug testing of clients, (c) regularly scheduled case reviews with a supervisor, (d) conducted case reviews by a quality review committee, (e) conducted outcome follow-up of discharged clients, (f) conducted periodic utilization review, and (g) conducted client satisfaction surveys. Each of these practices was scored 1 if the facility reported yes for the procedure and 0 if the facility reported no. This resulted in an additive scale ranging from 0 to 7.

Data analysis plan

All statistical analyses were conducted using IBM SPSS software (version 21.0). For the descriptive analysis we conducted cross-tabulations on the dependent variable (trauma services) with each of the demographic, population served, and organizational variables. The chi-square test ($p < .05$) was used to test for significant relationships between variables.

To determine if any of the independent variables were collinear, a zero-order correlation analysis was conducted on the interrelationships of all of the independent variables (not shown because of space considerations). None of the relationships exceeded $r = .50$, indicating that multicolinearity was not an issue.

For the multivariate analysis we conducted a step-wise binary logistic regression. In this analysis we regressed the dichotomous dependent variable (trauma services) on the demographic variables (Step 1), on the population served variables (Step 2), and then on the organizational variables (Step 3). This allowed us to assess the relative influence of each set of variables in predicting trauma services.

RESULTS

The results of the descriptive analyses are contained in Table 1. The findings indicate that overall approximately one fifth (19.6%) of outpatient substance abuse treatment programs provide trauma services. Region of the country was statistically significant, showing that fewer programs in the Midwest offered trauma services. There were no differences between urban and rural areas in the provision of trauma services.

All of the population served variables were significantly related to the provision of trauma services, with the strongest being veterans (34.6%),

TABLE 1 Characteristics of Outpatient Substance Abuse Treatment Facilities by the Availability of Trauma Services

	Trauma services			
	Never or rarely		Always or often	
Facility characteristics	*N*	%	*N*	%
Total	3,828	80.4	934	19.6
Region*				
Northeast	817	79.4	212	20.6
Midwest	934	83.0	191	17.0
South	1,008	80.8	240	19.2
West	1,069	78.6	291	21.4
Urbanicity				
Rural	1,924	80.9	454	19.1
Urban	1,904	79.9	480	20.1
Populations served				
Adolescents*	1,081	78.1	304	21.9
Cooccurring conditions*	938	69.5	411	30.5
Criminal justice*	906	77.2	268	27.8
Adult women*	1,225	71.0	500	29.0
Pregnant women*	552	72.6	208	27.4
Veterans*	149	65.4	79	34.6
Ownership*				
Not-for-profit	2,094	75.7	671	24.3
For profit	1,734	86.8	263	13.2
Size				
Small	1,546	79.4	401	20.6
Medium	721	79.6	185	20.4
Large	1,561	81.8	348	18.2
Uses sliding fee*	2,315	77.5	674	22.5
Offers free treatment*	1,527	74.7	518	25.3
Receives government funds*	1,918	75.0	638	25.0
Accreditation				
JCAHCO*	573	77.4	167	22.8
COA	149	77.2	44	22.8
Absorptive capacity*				
Low	852	89.8	97	10.2
High	2,976	78.0	837	22.0

Note: JCAHCO = Joint Commission on the Accreditation of Health Care Organizations; COA = Council on Accreditation.
$^{*}p < .05$.

people with cooccurring conditions (30.5%), adult women (29.0%), and pregnant women (27.4%).

The organizational variables that were significantly related to the provision of trauma services included ownership, financing, accreditation, and absorptive capacity. Not-for-profit agencies were more likely to provide trauma services (24.3% vs. 13.2%). Programs that used a sliding fee (22.5%), offered free treatment (25.3%), and received government funds (25.0%) were all more likely to provide trauma services. The facilities that reported being

TABLE 2 Logistic Regression of Trauma Services on Demographic, Populations Served, and Organizational Characteristics

	Step 1 OR	Step 2 OR	Step 3 OR
Region[a]			
Northeast	.951	.759*	.649*
Midwest	.773*	.796*	.613*
South	.898	.907	.812
Urbanicity	1.048*	1.047	1.062*
Populations served			
Adolescents		1.084	.963
Cooccurring		1.927*	1.844*
Criminal justice		.847	.809*
Adult women		2.024*	1.836*
Pregnant women		1.031	1.065
Veterans		1.388*	1.434*
Organizational characteristics			
Ownership			.766*
Size			.858*
Sliding fee			1.146
Free treatment			1.286*
Government funds			1.593*
Accreditation			
JCAHCO			1.310*
COA			1.095
Absorptive capacity			1.488*
Constant	.220*	.136*	.013*
Model chi-square	12.571*	230.059*	462.269*
Nagelkerke R^2	.004	.075	.147

Note: OR = odds ratio; JCAHCO = Joint Commission on the Accreditation of Health Care Organizations; COA = Council on Accreditation.
[a]For region the reference category is West.
*$p < .05$.

accredited by JCAHCO were more likely to provide trauma services (22.6%). Being accredited by COA was not significantly related to the provision of trauma services. Absorptive capacity was significantly related to the provision of trauma services; those that were high on absorptive capacity were more than twice as likely to provide trauma services (22.0% vs. 10.2%).

Table 2 contains the findings from the step-wise logistic regression analysis. On the first step, the demographic variables of region of the country and urbanicity were entered. The findings show that programs in the Midwest and those in more rural locations were less likely to offer trauma services. Although the model is statistically significant ($\chi^2 = 12.571$), it is not particularly strong (Nagelkerke $R^2 = .004$).

The second step included the demographic variables and the population served variables. The model is statistically significant ($\chi^2 = 230.089$) and explains approximately 7.5% of the variation in trauma services. The findings show that facilities that have programs dedicated to serving adult women are more than twice as likely to provide trauma services (OR = 2.024). The findings also show that facilities with programs specifically for people with cooccurring disorders (OR = 1.927) and programs for veterans (OR = 1.388) are also more likely to provide trauma services.

The final step in the analysis included adding the organizational variables. This step was statistically significant ($\chi^2 = 462.269$) and explains 14.7% of the variation in the provision of trauma services. The findings show that not-for-profit facilities are 24% more likely to provide trauma services (OR = .766) and that smaller programs are 15% more likely to provide trauma services (OR = .858). Facilities that offer free services are about 1.3 times more likely and those that accept government funds are 1.6 times more likely to provide trauma services. Facilities that are accredited by JCAHCO are 1.3 times more likely to provide trauma services. The findings related to absorptive capacity are quite strong: For every unit increase in absorptive capacity, there is a 48.8% increase in the probability of providing trauma care. Those facilities that score the highest on absorptive capacity are approximately 3.5 times more likely to provide trauma services than those that score at the lowest level of absorptive capacity.

Overall the findings from the final model confirmed most of the findings from the preliminary analyses. Facilities located in the West as compared to the Midwest and Northeast and those located in more urban areas are more likely to provide trauma services. Also, facilities that offer programs specifically for people with cooccurring conditions, women, and veterans are more likely to provide trauma-related services. Facilities that provide programs for criminal justice clients are less likely to provide trauma services.

DISCUSSION

There is convincing evidence of the cooccurrence of substance use disorders and trauma among treatment populations. In fact, 62% of substance abuse treatment facilities provide brief mental screenings that can be used to identify individuals in need of trauma services (SAMHSA Office of Applied Studies, 2010). However, only 19.7% of treatment facilities indicate that they "always" or "often" provide trauma services. It remains unclear why there is such low adoption of trauma services given the past two decades of research showing the high correlation between substance use disorders and trauma histories. Bride et al. (2011) noted that research on innovations in treatment for substance use disorders indicates that the adoption of such practices are often partially implemented focusing on specific subpopulations within the facility. This would seem to be supported by the results of this study that found programs that serve veterans, people with cooccurring disorders, and women were much more likely to provide trauma services.

Dass-Brailsford and Myrick (2010) identified a number of barriers that might limit the integration of trauma and substance abuse services. These include barriers at the clinical, organizational, and screening and assessment levels. Among the clinical barriers, the authors noted that clinicians might lack awareness of the role of trauma in the substance abuse treatment population and thus could fail to regularly screen or inadequately screen for trauma or PTSD (Ouimette, Brown, & Najavits, 1998; Read, Bollinger, & Sharkansky, 2003). Likewise, individuals seeking treatment might minimize symptoms to increase chances for treatment entry or to guard against other perceived discrimination. Finally, theoretical and philosophical approaches might view the substance use as the primary problem to be addressed and maintain that mental health issues such as trauma or PTSD should not be addressed until after abstinence is achieved (Brown, 2000).

From an organizational perspective, one possible explanation for the low level of adoption is the dearth of research about which models of integrated trauma treatment are most effective (Dass-Brailsford & Myrick, 2010). As a result, to recognize intervention services with a strong evidence base that can be implemented within a specific program or practice setting requires significant skills in terms of assessing cost, training requirements, fit with program and provider orientation, the setting, and the service population (SAMHSA, 2014). Organizations with limited resources and low absorptive capacity might not identify a need or a benefit in adopting trauma services or adopting a trauma-informed approach to care.

Another possible explanation for failure to adopt trauma services in outpatient substance abuse treatment might have to do with the program's organizational philosophy. Essentially, if the norms and values of the program establish the substance use disorder as the paramount problem, whether or not this view is endorsed by the clinical staff, abstinence could be viewed as the main clinical goal with cooccurring trauma issues as secondary (Harris & Fallot, 2001). If and when abstinence is achieved, the program could begin to address trauma as a recovery maintenance intervention or it might refer to a mental health facility.

The results also help provide additional insight into the way programs might have chosen to adopt trauma services. In this study, organizations that served individuals with cooccurring disorders, adult women, and veterans, who are often identified in the mainstream media as requiring PTSD treatment, were more likely to adopt trauma services. This could be a reflexive response by organizations that serve specific populations or, in some cases, a more proactive organizational strategy to develop services to target these specific populations. Consistent with previous research on characteristics of treatment, financing and accreditation were found to influence the adoption of trauma services. Programs that offered free treatment, received government funding, and met JCAHCO accreditation standards were more likely to provide trauma services. Here, the population served and organizational characteristics might be the prime influence on the values and norms of these organizations, which in turn could influence the receptivity of the organization and staff to adopt trauma services to meet the needs of the client population (Rogers, 2003).

Consistent with our expectations, organizations that regularly gathered and utilized information to assess program effectiveness were about one and a half times more likely to adopt trauma services than those that did not. One explanation is that organizations that have stronger communication ties with other organizations are exposed to more information regarding trauma, PTSD, and the cooccurrence of substance use disorders. As a result, these programs might be making treatment decisions based on information gathered from other substance abuse treatment agencies. Thus, increased absorptive capacity, defined as the ability of an organization to access and effectively use information, enhances the buy-in and cooperation of both management and clinical staff and could enhance overall implementation of services to address trauma and PTSD among their clients.

STUDY LIMITATIONS

In evaluating the results of this study, its limitations must be kept in mind. First, the information on organizational characteristics and services is based on self-report and is by its nature subject to reporting error. Second, the N-SSATS is a point-prevalence survey so certain characteristics such as facility size represent a snapshot of outpatient treatment facilities on a specific reference date rather than an annual average. Although the survey attempts to capture information from all known treatment facilities, it is voluntary, and does not adjust for the 7% facility nonresponse. Further, as noted earlier, the information about trauma services is limited to reported frequency of use and does not provide information on additional principles involved in many multidimensional definitions of trauma-informed care, the reasons for adopting or implementing models, or the extent of the populations that receive trauma services. Further research on the level of integration of trauma services into standard practice, including the level of training and sustained supervision, would help to illuminate the impact on values, norms, and implementation within treatment settings. Research that focuses on identifying the trauma-informed care models or elements of models that work best across a variety of organizational types is needed to help inform treatment programs' planning and strategies for implementation. Also, because the study was a secondary analysis of data, we were limited to what was asked in the original study. For example, factors related to workforce education and credentials (Knudsen & Roman, 2004), as well as caseload characteristics (Roman & Johnson, 2002), have been shown to be related to the adoption of innovations. We were not able to access data on these crucial factors.

IMPLICATIONS FOR SOCIAL WORK PRACTICE

Research that examines the administrative decisions that influence the motivation for offering trauma services in substance abuse treatment programs can lead to a better understanding of the role that absorptive capacity plays in identifying, adopting, and implementing innovative treatment protocols. It is important that new treatments not be implemented for implementation's sake, but that the decisions to adopt innovative services reflect the norms and values of the social work profession. This is clearly relevant for the implementation of trauma services.

Another area that warrants attention is the training of social work practitioners and managers who are on the front lines of treatment. Delany and colleagues (2009) noted that in the last two decades there has been increased attention to accountability in service organizations, resulting in increased emphasis on less intensive services and the adoption of interventions with a strong evidence base. This trend has not diminished under the Patient Portability and Affordable Care Act (ACA). The training of social workers to become trauma-informed providers of substance abuse treatment is critical for the further development of innovations in treatment. This training of social workers in trauma-informed care has the potential for positively impacting the program philosophies, and thus the treatment procedures of substance abuse treatment programs.

REFERENCES

Abraham, A. J., & Roman, P. M. (2010). Early adoption of injectable naltrexone for alcohol-use disorders: Findings in the private-treatment sector. *Journal of Studies on Alcohol and Drugs*, *71*, 460–466.

American Psychiatric Association. (1980). *Diagnostic and statistical manual of mental disorders* (3rd ed.). Washington, DC: Author.

Ball, S., Bachrach, K., DeCarlo, J., Farentinos, C., Keen, M., McSherry, T., . . . Carroll, K. (2002). Characteristics, beliefs and practices of community clinicians trained to provide manual-guided therapy for substance abusers. *Journal of Substance Abuse Treatment*, *23*, 309–318.

Bride, B. E., Abraham, A. J., & Roman, P. M. (2010). Diffusion of contingency management and attitudes regarding its effectiveness and acceptability. *Substance Abuse*, *31*, 127–135.

Bride, B. E., Abraham, A. J., & Roman, P. M. (2011). Organizational factors associated with the use of contingency management in publicly funded substance abuse treatment centers. *Journal of Substance Abuse Treatment*, *40*, 87–94.

Brown, P. J. (2000). Outcome in female patients with both substance use and post-traumatic stress disorders. *Alcoholism Treatment Quarterly*, *18*, 127–135.

Capezza, N. M., & Najavits, L. M. (2012). Rates of trauma-informed counseling at substance abuse treatment facilities: Reports from over 10,000 programs. *Psychiatric Services*, *63*, 390–394.

Crocq, D. F., & Crocq, M. A. (2000). From shell shock and war neurosis to post-traumatic stress disorder, *Psychoendricrinology*, *29*, 1281–1289.

Dass-Brailsford, P., & Myrick, A. C. (2010). Psychological trauma and substance abuse: The need for an integrated approach, *Trauma, Violence, & Abuse*, *11*, 202–213.

Davidson, J. R., Hughes, D. G., Blazer, D. G., & George, L. K. (1991). Post-traumatic stress disorder in the community: An epidemiological study. *Psychological Medicine. A Journal of Psychiatry and the Allied Sciences*, *21*, 713–721.

Delany, P. J., Shields, J. J., & Roberts, D. L. (2009). Program and client characteristics as predictors of the availability of community-based substance abuse treatment programs, *Journal of Behavioral Health Services and Research*, *36*, 450–464.

Ducharme, L. J., Knudsen, H. K., Roman, P. R., & Johnson, A. (2007). Innovation adoption in substance abuse treatment. Exposure, trialability, and the Clinical Trials Network. *Journal of Substance Abuse Treatment*, *32*, 321–329.

Farley, M., Golding, J. M., Young, G., Mulligan, M., & Minkoff, J. R. (2004). Trauma history and relapse probability among patients seeking substance abuse treatment. *Journal of Substance Abuse Treatment*, *27*, 161–167.

Fetzner, M. G., McMillan, K. A., Sareen, J., & Asmundson, G. J. (2011). What is the association between traumatic life events and alcohol abuse/dependence in people with and without PTSD? Findings from a nationally representative sample. *Depression and Anxiety*, *28*, 632–638.

Forman, R. F., Bovasso, G., & Woody, G. (2001). Staff beliefs about addiction treatment. *Journal of Substance Abuse Treatment*, *21*, 1–9.

Greenberg, G. A., & Rosenheck, R. A. (2010). Mental health correlates of past homelessness in the National Comorbidity Study Replication. *Journal of Health Care for the Poor and Underserved*, *21*, 1234–1249.

Harris, M., & Fallot, R. D. (Eds.). (2001). *Using trauma theory to design service systems: New directions for mental health services, No. 89*. San Francisco, CA: Jossey-Bass.

Holbrook, T. L., Hoyt, D. B., Stein, M. B., & Sieber, W. J. (2002). Gender differences in long-term posttraumatic stress disorder outcomes after major trauma: Women are at higher risk of adverse outcomes than men. *Journal of Trauma*, *53*, 882–888.

Ingram, D. D., & Franco, S. J. (2013). NCHS urban–rural classification scheme for counties. Atlanta, GA: National Center for Health Statistics.

Kessler, R. C., Sonnega, A., Bromet, A., Hughes, M., & Nelson, C. B. (1995). Posttraumatic-stress disorder in the national comorbidity survey. *Archives of General Pyschiatry*, *52*, 1048–1060.

Kimerling, R., Street, A. E., Pavao, J., Smith, M. W., Cronkite, R. C., Holmes, T. H., & Frayne, S. M. (2010). Military-related sexual trauma among veterans health administration patients returning from Afghanistan and Iraq. *American Journal of Public Health*, *100*, 1409–1412.

Knudsen, H. K., Ducharme, L. J., & Roman, P. M. (2006). Early adoption of buprenorphine in substance abuse treatment centers: Data from the private and public sectors. *Journal of Substance Abuse Treatment*, *30*, 363–373.

Knudsen, H. K., Ducharme, L. J., Roman, P. M., & Link, T. (2005). Buprenorphine diffusion: The attitudes of substance abuse treatment counselors. *Journal of Substance Abuse Treatment*, *29*, 95–106.

Knudsen, H. K., & Roman, P. M. (2004). Modeling the use of innovations in private treatment organizations: The role of absorptive capacity. *Journal of Substance Abuse Treatment*, *26*, 353–356.

Lamb, S., Greenlick, M. R., & McCarty, D. (Eds.). (1998). *Bridging the gap between research and practice: Forging partnerships with community-based drug and alcohol treatment, and practice: Forging partnerships with community-based drug and alcohol treatment*. Washington, DC: National Academies Press.

Liddle, H. A., Rowe, C. L., Quille, T. J., Dakof, G. A., Mills, D. S., Sakran, E., & Biaggi, H. (2002). Transporting a research-based adolescent treatment into practice. *Journal of Substance Abuse Treatment*, *22*, 231–243.

Martin, G. W., Herie, M. A., Turner, B. J., & Cunningham, J. A. (1998). A social marketing model for disseminating research-based treatments to addictions treatment providers. *Addiction*, *93*, 1703–1715.

Nickerson, A., Bryant, R. A., Silove, D., & Steel, Z. (2011). A critical review of psychological treatments of posttraumatic stress disorder in refugees, *Clinical Psychology Review*. *31*, 399–417.

Olf, M., Langeland, W., Draijer, N., & Gersons, B. P. (2007). Gender differences in posttraumatic stress disorder. *Psychological Bulletin*, *133*, 183–204.

Ouimette, P. C., Brown, P. J., & Najavits, L. M. (1998). Course and treatment of patients with both substance use and post-traumatic stress disorders. *Addictive Behaviors*, *23*, 785–795.

Petersilia, J. R. (2001). Crime victims with developmental disabilities: A review essay. *Criminal Justice and Behavior*, *28*(6), 655–694.

Pole, N., Gone, J. P., & Kulkarni, M. (2008). Post-traumatic stress disorder among ethnoracial minorities in the United States. *Clinical Psychology: Science and Practice*, *15*, 35–61.

Pratchett, L. C., Pelcovitz, M. R., & Yehuda, R. (2010). Trauma and violence: Are women the weaker sex? *Psychiatric Clinics of North America*, *33*, 465–474.

Read, J. P., Bollinger, A. R., & Sharkansky, E. J. (2003). Assessment and diagnosis of PTSD-substance abuse. In P. C. Ouimette & P. Brown (Eds.), *Trauma and substance abuse: Causes, consequences, and the treatment of co-morbidity* (pp. 111–125). Washington, DC: American Psychological Association.

Roberts, A. L., Gilman, S. E., Breslau, J., Breslau, N., & Koenen, K. C. (2011). Race/ethnic differences in exposure to traumatic events, development of post-traumatic stress disorder, and treatment-seeking for post-traumatic stress disorder in the United States. *Psychological Medicine*, *41*, 71–83.

Rogers, E. M. (2003). *Diffusion of innovations* (5th ed.). New York, NY: Free Press.

Roman, P. M., & Johnson, J.A. (2002). Adoption and implementation of new technologies in substance abuse treatment. *Journal of Substance Abuse Treatment*, *22*, 211–218.

Rosenheck, R. (2001). Stages in the implementation of innovative clinical programs in complex organizations. *Journal of Nervous and Mental Disease*, *189*, 812–821.

Simpson, D.D. (2002). A conceptual framework for transferring research to practice. *Journal of Substance Abuse Treatment*, *22*, 171–182.

Substance Abuse and Mental Health Services Administration. (2013a). *National Survey of Substance Abuse Treatment Services (N-SSATS): 2012. Data on substance abuse treatment facilities* (BHSIS Series S-66, HHS Publication No. [SMA] 14-4809). Rockville, MD: Author.

Substance Abuse and Mental Health Services Administration. (2013b). *Results from the 2012 National Survey on Drug Use and Health* (NSDUH Series H-46, HHS Publication No. [SMA] 13-4795). Rockville, MD: Author.

Substance Abuse and Mental Health Services Administration. (2014). *Trauma-informed care in behavioral health services* (Treatment Improvement Protocol [TIP] Series 57, HHS Pub. No. [SMA] 13-4801). Rockville, MD: Author.

Substance Abuse and Mental Health Services Administration Office of Applied Studies. (2010, September 30). *The N-SSATS Report: Mental health screenings and trauma-related counseling in substance abuse treatment facilities*. Rockville, MD: Author.

Truman, J. L. (2011). *Crime victimization, 2010* (NCJ 235508). Washington, DC: U.S. Department of Justice.

Van der Kolk, B. A. (2007). The history of trauma in psychiatry. In M. J. Friedman, T. M. Keane, & P. A. Resick (Eds.), *Handbook of PTSD: Science & practice* (pp. 19–33). New York, NY: Guilford.

Trauma-Informed Care and Addiction Recovery: An Interview With Nancy J. Smyth, PhD, LCSW

INTERVIEW CONDUCTED BY
LORI HOLLERAN STEIKER, MSW, PHD
Associate Professor, School of Social Work, University of Texas at Austin, Austin, Texas, USA

Holleran Steiker: It is a privilege to interview the Dean of the School of Social Work at the State University of New York at Buffalo. You wear a number of hats: dean, professor, researcher, and clinician. You are a Board Certified Expert in Traumatic Stress through the American Academy of Experts in Traumatic Stress and have worked in both mental health and addiction-treatment settings for over 35 years as a clinician, manager, educator, researcher, and program developer. To begin with, can you tell us about trauma-informed care and what brought you to study this area?

Smyth: I'll start with the second part of the question and come back to the first. I got my start in social work working with people who had severe mental illness during the 1980s and then moved into working with people who were struggling with alcohol and other drug problems. In both groups of people I was struck by the high prevalence of significant trauma histories, both in childhood and adulthood. For this reason, I began educating myself about the impact of trauma and its treatment. As I learned more I also recognized the importance of listening to the experiences of trauma survivors themselves, including their negative experiences in our systems of care. Stories like that of Anna—a young woman with a history of sexual abuse and a diagnosis of schizophrenia who had the treatment system fail her, despite good intentions (Jennings, 1994)—made it clear that sometimes our service systems inadvertently harmed clients by re-creating aspects of their traumatic experiences or reinforcing the negative beliefs about themselves that originated in their traumatic experiences. Bloom and Farragher (2011) recently described these negative system effects on both clients and staff in their book, *Destroying Sanctuary*.

For all of the above reasons, trauma-informed care (TIC) was identified as a priority by the Substance Abuse and Mental Health Services Administration (SAMHSA) and they created the National Center for Trauma-Informed Care (NCTIC) in 2005 through a shared initiative with the National Association of State Mental Health Program Directors (SAMHSA, 2014). Simply stated, TIC is an approach to designing policy, systems of care, and our clinical practice based on what we know from research about the impact of trauma on people, as well the knowledge from our research that most of the clients in our service systems have had significant exposure to traumatic events over the course of their lives (Smyth & Greyber, 2013). Recognizing that traumatic events made people feel unsafe and powerless, TIC seeks to ensure that clients and staff feel safe and empowered, and is organized around the principles of safety/trustworthiness, choice/collaboration/empowerment, and a strengths-based approach (Hopper, Bassuk, & Olivet, 2010).

At the practice level, TIC asks "What happened to you?" versus "What's wrong with you?" and, therefore incorporates the assessment of trauma and trauma symptoms routinely into all practice approaches. However, this is done by allowing the client to control the pace of disclosure, as well as by ensuring that clients leave the office feeling calm and contained should such disclosures be upsetting. TIC also ensures that clients have access to trauma-focused (sometimes called trauma-specific) interventions; that is, interventions that treat the consequences of traumatic stress.

TIC focuses our attention on the ways in which services are delivered and service systems are organized (Bloom & Farragher, 2011). Trauma-informed organizations ensure that every staff member, from the receptionist to the executive director, understands trauma and trauma reactions. Trauma-informed organizations routinely examine all policies, procedures, and processes to ensure they are not likely to trigger trauma reactions or to be experienced as retraumatizing; that is, putting a client through a process that shares characteristics of the traumas he or she has lived through. An example of such a retraumatizing process would be pushing a client to disclose a rape experience in group therapy before she or he feels ready to do so. Such an experience is reminiscent of the powerless and vulnerability of the rape itself—I've seen too many clients drop out of substance abuse treatment after an experience just like this.

Holleran Steiker: Can you give us an overview of evidence-based trauma interventions and their particular utility?

Smyth: One challenge in interpreting the effectiveness of most of our trauma treatment methods is that the treatment research studies focus on diagnosis, such as posttraumatic stress disorder (PTSD), not on clients having had the experience of trauma. Not all clients who experience trauma develop PTSD. Research indicates that traumatic experiences can result in a range of psychiatric symptoms, not just PTSD (see, e.g., Ross, 2011).

There are several evidence-based treatments for PTSD. There is significant evidence to support the effectiveness of cognitive behavior therapy for PTSD among adults, most specifically, prolonged exposure and then cognitive processing treatment (Friedman, Cohen, Foa, & Keane, 2009). In addition, eye movement desensitization and reprocessing (EMDR) is also considered an effective treatment for treating PTSD in adults (Friedman et al, 2009). Among children and adolescents, the treatment with the most research support is trauma-focused cognitive-behavior therapy (Friedman et al, 2009).

However, it's important to note that the empirical support for the previously mentioned treatments did not evaluate these treatments on people with coexisting PTSD and substance use disorders. A review of the evidence for these treatments indicates that *Seeking Safety* (Najavits & Hein, 2013; Najavits et al., 2009) has the most support in treating this population—most of the studies have been done on adults.

Holleran Steiker: What are the basic assumptions of trauma-informed care for people with substance use disorders?

Smyth: The basic assumptions are the same as for all clients. However, it's helpful to remember some of these wise words from clients. To paraphrase many of the clients I worked with over the years, "Initially, alcohol and other drugs saved my life, then, later, they turned on me"—by that, clients mean that they often started using very young, after living through their own versions of hell, and substances allowed them to continue to face living their lives. In my experience, clients won't be able to achieve successful, sustained recovery without learning new skills to deal with their feelings in their day-to-day lives. Seeking Safety (Najavits, 2002, 2014) is one such treatment that provides these skills. But that, by itself, is not trauma-informed care. Trauma-informed care will provide Seeking Safety in a setting that provides safety, trustworthiness, empowerment, choice, and collaboration with clients and with staff. The latter element is an important focus in trauma-informed care.

I generally think of treatments for trauma in two broad categories: those that help clients manage their emotions, their triggers (for substance use and for trauma symptoms), and their lives without turning to risky behaviors that place them in more danger (e.g., substance use, self-injury, dissociation, and unsafe sexual behaviors); and those that help them emotionally process and integrate traumatic memories. The former I call *stabilization treatments,* the latter, *emotional processing treatments*. One best practice that I've found to be important is that the clients need to have the tools to manage their emotions and triggers for substance use and for trauma symptoms before treatment can focus on emotionally processing the traumatic memories themselves. In other words, stabilization treatments come first, then, when the client is ready (and willing), emotional processing treatments are appropriate, with a return to a focus on stabilization whenever the client appears to need it. This approach is generally consistent with treating many populations who require a more sequenced approach for the treatment of their trauma (Courtois & Ford, 2009).

Holleran Steiker: Your research, teaching, and practice all hone in on trauma, substance abuse, and on working with people recovering from those experiences. What are the innovations for social workers in the field (e.g., EMDR and mindfulness meditation)? And please elaborate on how one gets trained to utilize these techniques.

Smyth: There are many exciting developments in new treatments for trauma, as well as treatments for coexisting disorders of trauma and substance abuse. Dialectical behavior therapy (DBT, which uses mindfulness training), although not developed as a trauma treatment, is often now used by practitioners as a stabilization treatment with people with both disorders. Using DBT effectively requires extensive training and consultation (see http://behavioraltech.org/). Other treatments that one hears more about these days are mindfulness mediation or mindfulness-based stress reduction, sensorimotor body processing, yoga, thought-field therapy, neurofeedback, acceptance and commitment therapy—the list goes on and on. Honestly, though, this is not where I would start with treatment, because I think one has to have a solid sense for what is achievable with research-supported treatments before one can reasonably evaluate the contribution of the newer treatments. In addition, clients still don't have consistent access to the treatments that have research support—my own bias is that clients have a right to have access to these research-based treatments first and foremost—then value might be added by bringing in some of the newer treatment options. Access to evidence-based trauma treatments also is a fundamental part of trauma-informed care.

The best strategy for to obtaining training in specific treatment methods is to contact the treatment developer or an organization responsible for certifying practitioners. For prolonged exposure, contact Edna Foa (http://www.med.upenn.edu/ctsa/); for cognitive processing therapy, Patricia Resick or https://www.newpaltz.edu/idmh/idmh_cpt_training.pdf; and for EMDR, Francine Shapiro or the EMDR International Association (www.emdria.org). The National Child Traumatic Stress Network offers a web-based training in trauma-focused cognitive behavior therapy that has been evaluated primarily for use with children and adolescents and can be found at http://www.nctsn.org/products/nctsn-affiliated-resources/tf-cbt-web.

I also recommend that practitioners join national professional organizations, such as the International Association for Traumatic Stress Studies (www.istss.org) and the International Society for the Study of Trauma and Dissociation (www.isst-d.org). Both are good sources for staying up-to-date on trauma treatment methods and both offer training on trauma treatment. The latter offers an online training course in treating dissociation, a knowledge area that I have found to be very important in treating people with coexisting trauma and substance use disorders.

Holleran Steiker: Can you explain the existing efforts, settings, unmet needs, and related challenges with regard to trauma-informed care when working with clients with substance use disorders?

Smyth: Anecdotally, I've seen more substance use disorder treatment settings embrace a TIC model of treatment in recent years. Some of the challenges they face are the traditional substance use treatment approach that minimizes client choice and collaboration, especially in the early stages of treatment. If motivational interviewing has been embraced by treatment programs, then TIC is a more natural "fit." Another challenge is that TIC would allow clients to take a harm reduction approach to their treatment and come to their own conclusions about whether or not they need to be totally abstinent, and yet in some states, treatment program regulations might not allow this as a valid option within a treatment program. Even so, I've seen treatment programs find creative ways to use treatment plan documentation to find a way around this requirement. A third challenge I've seen arise is when a criminal justice professional working with a client refuses to let the treatment professionals take a trauma-informed approach. This highlights the need for training within the criminal justice system, a priority that SAMHSA has adopted—I know that our Institute on Trauma and Trauma-Informed Care has had some significant success in providing training for criminal justice professionals in our region (Finkle, 2014).

Holleran Steiker: Will you tell some anecdotes as illustrations of your experiences, successes, or challenges with trauma-informed care with people struggling with substance use disorders or in recovery?

Smyth: Trauma-informed care recognizes the importance of trust in treatment. It also recognizes that practitioners have power over clients and that most of our clients have been hurt by people in authority who were supposed to be trustworthy and weren't, therefore trusting is that much harder for them. For this reason, I start treatment by explaining to my clients that if they are like many of the people I have seen, they have many good reasons not to trust people. For this reason I want us to take the time to make sure they know what they can expect from me in terms of my role and availability, and, of course, any limits to confidentiality. I then tell them not to trust me until they have tested my trustworthiness and we rehearse how they can let me know they don't want to talk about something. We then explore how they might test my (and other people's) trustworthiness. Paradoxically, this whole focus often engenders some trust, because it gives the client the power to set the pace for trusting. However, trust can take a long time to build, and it has many layers. In the case of clients who were abused or abandoned by their therapists, sometimes it can take years before they can begin to trust that I won't do the same to them.

All the clients I've worked with believe that they are broken, that they are fundamentally not "fixable." I start by educating them on how trauma, especially childhood trauma, shapes that belief, especially the feeling of shame—and that, in reality, the feeling of shame belongs to the perpetrator, not to them, even though it doesn't feel that way. We then talk about how, in adulthood, the relapse they experience during their addiction—often caused by feelings of shame—just confirms in their minds that they are fundamentally broken and won't be able to be successful in recovery. Most clients won't be able to develop sustained recovery without addressing their core belief about being broken, and this will need to be achieved by emotional processing trauma treatment (also called trauma processing). However, few people want to do that treatment, because it means going back over very painful experiences. Often clients will insist that they can stay sober using all the tools of stabilization treatment and self-help groups and that they don't need to do the trauma-processing treatment.

Trauma-informed care leaves the choice about whether or not to do the trauma-processing treatment with the client. So for clients who refuse to accept the need to do trauma processing, we work closely together to help them strengthen their stabilization skills, and we do relapse prevention treatment with the use of solution-focused questions. For example, I might ask, "How will you know when it's time to work on the memories of the trauma? What will you be doing? What will you be feeling?" I then have the client imagine such a moment and then see themselves reaching out for help at that time, instead of giving in to hopelessness and reaching for some way to hurt or kill themselves. After doing this, I have had more than one person show up back in treatment, often many months or years later, when the moment we had rehearsed actually happened, seeking help as an alternative to suicide. Preparing and waiting for such moments can be scary for the practitioner. For this reason, I can't emphasize enough the importance of good supervision or consultation.

Holleran Steiker: What are your visions for this area of work and study in the future?

Smyth: Research tells us that all human services programs have clients with significant trauma histories (Smyth & Greyber, 2013). As a result, I hope to see TIC adopted by more and more agencies and, finally, entire service systems. This is the reason that at the University at Buffalo we have transformed our master's in social work (MSW) curriculum so that every student learns TIC in addition to all the other skills and knowledge that one picks up in an MSW program.

Although the anecdotal evidence we've received from agencies who have adopted this approach has been very encouraging, I would like to see more research done on treatment outcomes and staff retention and wellness. To do such research well, we need to be able to assess the degree to which an agency is implementing a TIC model. Our Institute on Trauma and Trauma-Informed Care has been working with other experts to develop and test tools that will help agencies do this.

Holleran Steiker: What recommendations can you make to social workers who want to create, aid, or research trauma-informed care for people with substance use disorders in their agencies and communities?

Smyth: Begin by getting training and consultation on TIC and by linking to others who are using these approaches. A good Google search on trauma-informed care and on trauma will reveal many good resources. I also have a list of other resources you can learn more from in a recent blog post (Smyth, 2013) that I wrote about this topic. However, it's helpful to find a structured continuing education program to take you through the basics. The National Center for Trauma-Informed Care (SAMHSA, 2014) is a good place to start, as is the National Child Traumatic Stress Network (NCTSN, 2014). We have an online trauma-informed care training program (http://socialwork.buffalo.edu/continuing-education/certificate-programs/trauma.html), and our Institute on Trauma and Trauma-Informed Care has been successful helping agencies access some grant money to bring the training to their staff.

Once you have grounding in TIC, begin obtaining some solid training and consultation in stabilization treatments—Seeking Safety (Najavits, 2014) is a great place to start. Beyond the training, it's critical to get good consultation and supervision. A good way to cut costs for this is to team up with others who want to learn, either within your agency, or through creating a small group that consults with an expert via telephone conferencing or an encrypted web-conferencing software program. You can share costs and learn from each other's cases. Training in emotional processing treatments should only follow after one has established a firm foundation in trauma-informed care and stabilization treatments.

Holleran Steiker: Can our readers contact you if they would like to learn more? If so, what is the best way to reach you?

Smyth: I would encourage readers to first contact our Institute on Trauma and Trauma-Informed Care (socialwork.buffalo.edu/ittic) because they are my "go-to" people on this topic. In conjunction with our continuing education department, they have been training many different service providers in this important model of care. However, if readers want to contact me, the best way to do so is through e-mail (sw-dean@buffalo.edu) or, even better, Twitter (@njsmyth).

REFERENCES

Bloom, S. L., & Farragher, B. (2011). *Destroying sanctuary: The crisis in human services delivery systems.* New York, NY: Oxford University Press.

Courtois, C. A., & Ford, J. D. (Eds.). (2009). *Treating complex traumatic stress disorders: An evidence-based guide.* New York, NY: Guilford.

Finkle, E. (2014, September 24). Trauma-informed judges take gentler approach, administer problem-solving justice to stop cycle of ACES. Retrieved from http://acestoohigh.com/2014/09/24/trauma-informed-judges-take-gentler-approach-administer-problem-solving-justice-to-stop-cycle-of-aces/

Friedman, M. J., Cohen, J. A., Foa, E. B., & Keane, T. M. (2009). Integration and summary. In E. B. Foa, T. M. Keane, M. J. Friedman, & J. A. Cohen (Eds.), *Effective treatments for PTSD: Practice guidelines from the International Society for Traumatic Stress Studies* (2nd ed., pp. 617–642). New York, NY: Guilford.

Hopper, E. K., Bassuk, E. L., & Olivet, J. (2010). Shelter from the storm: Trauma-informed care in homelessness services. *The Open Health Services and Policy Journal, 3*, 80–100. Retrieved from http://homeless.samhsa.gov/ResourceFiles/cenfdthy.pdf

Institute on Trauma and Trauma-Informed Care. (2014). Institute on Trauma and Trauma-Informed Care. Retrieved from www.socialwork.buffalo.edu/ittic

Jennings, A. (1994). On being invisible in the mental health system. *Journal of Behavioral Health Services and Research, 21*, 374–387. Retrieved from www.theannainstitute.org/obi.html

Najavits, L. M. (2002). *Seeking Safety: A treatment manual for PTSD and substance abuse.* New York, NY: Guilford.

Najavits, L. M. (2014). *Seeking Safety: A model to improve coping skills.* Retrieved from www.seekingsafety.org

Najavits, L. M., & Hein, D. (2013). Helping vulnerable populations: A comprehensive review of the treatment outcome literature on substance use disorder and PTSD. *Journal of Clinical Psychology, 69*, 433–479.

Najavits, L. M., Ryngala, D., Back, S. E., Bolton, E., Mueser, K. T., & Brady, K. T. (2009). Comorbid disorders. In E. B. Foa, T. M. Keane, M. J. Friedman, & J. A. Cohen (Eds.), *Effective treatments for PTSD: Practice guidelines from the International Society for Traumatic Stress Studies* (2nd ed., pp. 508–535). New York, NY: Guilford.

National Child Traumatic Stress Network. (2014). National Child Traumatic Stress Network. Retrieved from http://www.nctsnet.org/

Ross, C. A. (2011). *The trauma model: A solution to the problem of comorbidity in psychiatry*. Austin, TX: Greenleaf Book Group.

Smyth, N. J. (2013, April 19). Trauma-informed social work practice: What is it and why should we care? [Blog post]. Retrieved from http://njsmyth.wordpress.com/2013/04/19/trauma-informed-social-work-practice/

Smyth, N. J., & Greyber, L. (2013). Trauma-informed practice. In B. A. Thyer, C. N. Dulmus, & K. M. Sowers (Eds.), *Developing evidence-based generalist practice skills* (pp. 25–50). Hoboken, NJ: Wiley.

Substance Abuse and Mental Health Services Administration. (2014). National Center for Trauma-Informed Care. Retrieved from http://www.samhsa.gov/nctic/about

A Place in the World

KIMBERLY D. HONAKER, BA
Research Coordinator, Morgantown, West Virginia, USA

> As I began to love myself I recognized that my mind can disturb me and it can make me sick. But as I connected it to my heart, my mind became a valuable ally.
>
> —Charles Chaplin

I stood outside the Monongahela building, pacing back and forth before stepping across the threshold to hit the 8 button on an elevator that would take me to my therapists' floor. I didn't know what was happening to me. Six months sober, not a drop, and I had had a blackout. A blackout! No memory of the past 2 days and a slew of receipts for clothes that didn't resemble anything close to what I considered "my style" hanging neatly in the bedroom closet. I searched all the usual hiding places: atop the quilt basket collecting dust in the attic, beneath a row of carefully stacked toilet paper in the hall closet, all the dark corners of the basement, and my favorite, the space in the trunk where my spare tire was supposed to fit snugly. But they all came up empty. There were no "empties," no evidence of a binge in sight, no hangover even, yet something was missing. I was missing: for 2 whole days.

When my therapist opened the door and ushered me in, I couldn't make eye contact. I was ashamed of a drunk I didn't remember, and terrified of what else might have happened. As we began reconstructing the events that led up to my exit of 48 hours, I became more and more frightened. Was I demon possessed? Did someone kidnap me? "Whiteouts" I called them, like the old eraser tool on the typewriter page, my memory of what happened, disappeared.

I had previously attributed these missing-in-action moments to intoxication, and even though I began drinking at an early age, the 17-year span from birth through high school left too many moments of my life unaccounted for.

My sobriety began in January 1990. I was attending several 12-step meetings a week, hanging out with new friends in recovery, and trying not to separate from the thin tether of hope that kept me going back to therapy and to Alcoholics Anonymous (AA). The literature on trauma and addiction was scarce. Many addiction treatment professionals and programs offered this advice: Work on getting sober and clean first, then you can focus on your trauma. No one could answer the question: "What happens when your trauma focuses on you?"

As my therapist, Evelyn, and I began to uncover the sequences of my life, I raged. I raged that alcohol was no longer able to cut me free from my past. I raged at the unbearable truths beginning to surface in my sessions. I would sit mute, unable to speak, for moments on end. I argued with her about posttraumatic stress disorder. That's not what is wrong with me! I have an adjustment disorder! There were times, too, when I didn't even know how I got to her office. But fortunately for me, a few things remained steadfast: I knew that she was listening and would not disappear, even if I did for a while. I knew that she could bear to hear my losses and be my witness. I needed a witness. I needed to know I was not a ghost.

So many parallels, so many things that trip the memory switch. Without alcohol I was unable to stop the current of sounds, smells, images, and ache. I didn't know how to survive. But my therapist knew. She knew and lent me power with this pronouncement: "Kimberly, you survived the first time and I believe you will get through." No fancy terminology, no textbook cases to prove her "belief," but I held onto her words, and they became my mantra: "Evelyn believes I will survive. Evelyn says I *did* survive."

Recovery from trauma is a lot like grief, I think. Everyone has a different tale and a way they got there, but in the beginning there is this terrible, terrible loss. This is true, too, of addiction. The grief I felt over losing the ability to get drunk, over losing some perceived control by "disappearing," over trying to fit into a sober suit in a drunken world, made me sad beyond belief. At 27, I started to grieve; I started to grieve my whole life.

The trajectory of my therapy and my recovery looks something like this: remembering, forgetting, getting lost, coming back, holding on, letting go, coming to believe, disavowing that belief, deciding at last that I am a human being, deciding I am allowed to walk upright on the planet. The order of these events was unpredictable, but I was fortunate enough to have a very predictable therapist. A therapist who asked these important questions: "Where did you go? How did you get back?" and affirmed: "I'm so glad you're back, I'm so glad you survived." When I questioned that, she'd say, "You're sitting here, aren't you, Kimberly?"

There were a lot of times I wanted to drink, badly, but I knew the blackouts couldn't compete with the "whiteouts." I knew that eventually I would not be able to get drunk enough or stay drunk enough to disappear. Because some part of me decided to quit drinking, some part of me was going to AA, and some part of me was sitting there, with my therapist, grieving all the parts that didn't make it back.

After 5 years, a series of hard sessions, and much steadfast support, Evelyn retired. There have been times since I have needed help to remember that I am not a ghost. This past January I celebrated 24 years of sobriety and I have been recovering from trauma since 6 months past the day I got sober, until now. There have been long stretches of my life I wasn't sure I wanted to be here. There have also been long stretches of my life filled with contentment, accomplishment, and awe. I am not "recovered" exactly, but I do claim this: I honor my past, I honor my present, and I am grateful for a shot at the future.

Near the end of our time together, my last therapist, Katie, smiled, looked up at me, and spoke these words: "I am glad you are on the planet, Kimberly." The echo of Evelyn's voice hit every note inside me: I am still alive, I am still sober, and I have a witness, a few of them, to prove it.

I am grateful for you, my helpers, for your ability to translate this map of my life into a language I can speak, and call my own. Never underestimate the power of your words, the privilege of your client's trust, and the steadfast place you hold in the world. Not just your client's world, but your own. Look around, claim your spot. You got here, didn't you? I'm so glad you did.

Index

Note: Page numbers in *italics* represent tables
Page numbers in **bold** represent figures

Abraham, A.: Roman, P. and Bride, B. 117
absorptive capacity concept 117
abuse 8, 26–7, 72; adult 10; assessment 30–1; childhood 8, 26, 44–61, 91; and drug use 45–6; emotional 27–32, 35–7, 45, 68; and gender correlation 45–7, 56, 59; and neglect 27–30, 33, 36–7, 72; physical 8, 27–32, 45, 68, 72; substance 7, 45, 91, 114–18, 124, 138, *see also* sexual abuse
acute stress disorder 2
Adams, S.: Leukefeld, C. and Peden, A. 47
Adlaf, E.: and Breslin, F. 83
Adoption and Safe Families Act (ASFA, 1997) 19; and court-order reunification 19–20
adult abuse 10
adverse childhood experiences (ACE): and drug courts study 3, 44–61
Adverse Childhood Experiences study 45
age 50, 71
aggression 27
agoraphobia 50; drug courts study 54–5, 58
alcohol 13, 29, 92; dependence 45, 49, 52–3; and homeless youth study 66–85; rates 15
alcohol use disorder 31, 34, 75–9
Alcohol Use Disorders and Associated Disabilities Interview Schedule (AUDADIS) 29–30
Alcoholics Anonymous (AA) 144–5
ambiguous loss 9–11, 20; impacts 9
American Academy of Experts in Traumatic Stress 134
American Psychiatric Association (APA) 1–2, 25, 49, 116
amphetamines 75
antisocial personality disorder 69
anxiety 2, 44, 49; disorders 29–36; drug courts study 49, 54–5, 58–60
assault 68, 82; sexual 91
avoidance behaviors 50, 82

Beck Anxiety Inventory (BAI) 49–50, 53–5
Beck Depression Inventory-II (BDI) 49–50, 53–5
behaviors: avoidance 50, 82; criminal/deviant 69; sexual risk 12–13
Birkett, M.: Espelage, D. and Koenig, B. 103
Black, D.: *et al.* 27
Bloom, S.: and Farragher, B. 135
Bonferroni, C.E. 51–6
Bontempo, D.: and D'Augelli, A. 104
bootstrapping 51, 55
border rights 20
Boyle, T. 103
Breslin, F.: and Adlaf, E. 83
Bride, B.: Abraham, A. and Roman, P. 117; *et al.* 115, 123
bulimia 49, 54–5, 58
bullying 91

cannabis 49
Capezza, N.: and Najavits, L. 115
care: foster 11; health 19; prenatal 10; trauma-informed (TIC) 4, 47–8, 134–41
Census Bureau (US) 29
Centers for Disease Control (CDCs) 26, 91

Chaplin, C. 143
Chemtob, C.: *et al.* 10
child mortality rate 11
child protection 20; orders 16
Child Protective Services (CPS) 14–18
Child Welfare League of America 19
child welfare services 11, 19
childbearing 10
childhood 3; adverse experiences and gambling 25–38; death 12; parental difficulties exposure 14–16; sexual abuse (CSA) and drug courts study 44–61; welfare systems 11
Childhood Trauma Questionnaire (CTQ) 30, 72
cocaine 10, 49, 52–3, 67, 75
cognitive-behavioral therapy (CBT) 116, 136–7
commitment therapy 137
community 12
comparative fit index (CFI) 51, 57
competence 69–70, 74
Comprehensive Assessment for Drug Involved Women (CADIW) 13–14
confidentiality 20–1, 139
Conflict Tactics Scale (CTS) 30
Conroy, E.: *et al.* 45
contingency management 115
coping: and healing treatments 19–21
coping mechanisms 47, 50, 60, 69; avoidance 69, 73, 79; problem-focused 69–70, 73–4; social 74, 79, 83
Coping Scale 73
Council on Accreditation (COA) 120–2
counseling: trauma-related 119
courts: drug and childhood sexual abuse (CSA) 44–61
criminal history 50–1, 72, 82; behavior 69; and drug courts study 51–2, *52*
criminal justice system 18, 138; and court costs 26

Dass-Brailsford, P.: and Myrick, A. 124
D'Augelli, A.: and Bontempo, D. 104
dealing: drugs 68–9, 72, 82
death 2, 9; childhood 12; impact 9; threatened 2
debt 26
Delany, P.: Smith, K. and Shields, J. 3, 114–29
delinquency 11
depression 2, 44, 49, 53-5, 58-60, 69, 95
Destroying Sanctuary (Bloom and Farragher) 135
deviant behavior 69
Diagnostic and Statistical Manual of Mental Disorders (DSM-5) 1–2, 8, 25, 30, 116; and PDSQ Axis I disorders instrument 49–50; Task Force 1
dialectical behavior therapy (DBT) 137
differences: ethnic intergenerational 10–11
disclosure-related trauma 105
discrimination 124
disenfranchisement 9
disrupted mothering 18–19
dissociation 2, 47
distress: psychological 95–6, *97–8*, 103–5, 115
divorce 26–8, 32
Dore, P.: Elze, D. and Stiffman, A. 103–4
Driving While Intoxicated (DWI) 50–2
drug use 3, 11–13, 49; and abuse 45–6; and dealing 68–9, 72, 82; and homeless youth study 66–85; illicit 9–10; prescription 75
drug use disorder 31, 34, 79–81, *80*; model 79, *80*
Ducharme, L.: Roman, P. and Knudsen, H. 117
dummy coding 72
Dunlap, S.: Goldbach, J. and Fisher, B. 3, 90–113
Duran, B.: Duran, E. and Yellow Horse Brave Heart, M. 8

EBSCO Academic databases 92
ecstasy 75
education 13–18, 31–2, 50; sexual 12; status 72, 75; vocational skills 18
Elze, D.: Stiffman, A. and Dore, P. 103–4
emotional abuse 27–32, 35–7, 45, 68
emotional neglect 27–9
emotional processing treatments 137
employment 13, 18; illegal 68, 72, 82; as protective factor 69, 73; status 50
Espelage, D.: *et al.* 103–4; Koenig, B. and Birkett, M. 103
ethnicity 10–13, 50, 71, 75, 116

eye movement desensitization and reprocessing (EMDR) 116, 136, 137

Fallot, R.: and Harris, M. 116
family: LGB support and rejection 95, *98–9*, 103–5, 108; resilience 12
Family Acceptance Project 108
Farragher, B.: and Bloom, S. 135
Farrell, M.: Wolf, M. and Nochajski, T. 3, 44–65
Felsher, J.: *et al.* 27–8
Fisher, B.: Dunlap, S. and Goldbach, J. 3, 90–113
Flewelling, R.: Paschall, M. and Ringwalt, C. 83
Foa, E. 137
foster care 11
Future Time Perspective Scale (FTP) 74

gambling 72; and adverse childhood experiences study 3, 25–38; assessment 30; pathological disorder (PGD) 25–8; pathways model/groups 28; problem (PG) 25–8; risk factors 28–9; societal cost 26; Veteran's Administration treatment program 27
Gambling Impact and Behavior Study 26
Gay Straight Alliance 103–4
Gazel, R.: Rickman, D. and Thompson, W. 26
gender 10–11, 50, 71, 116; and abuse correlation 45–7, 56, 59; intergenerational differences 10–11; -specific sexual health 12; and substance use 45
genocide 8–9
Goldbach, J.: Fisher, B. and Dunlap, S. 3, 90–113
Grant, B.: Harford, T. and Yi, H. 27
grief 8, 19, 106, 144–5; child death 12; disenfranchized 9
guilt 9

hallucinogens 67, 75
Harford, T.: *et al.* 30–1; Yi, H. and Grant, B. 27
Harris, M.: and Fallot, R. 116
hate crimes 91
healing: cultural centers 19; treatments 19–21
health 12; care 19; cultural centers 19–20; mental 12, 28, 32–6, 49, 58, 124; poor self-rated 26; public 91; sexual 12
Healthy People 2020 program 91–2
Hein, D.: and Najavits, L. 136
Hepatitis 12
heroin 16, 49, 52–3, 67, 75
HerStory to Health project 12–21
HIV/AIDS 12, 105
Hodgins, D.: *et al.* 27
Holleran Steiker, L. 4, 134–42
homophobia 96, 104
Honaker, K. 4, 143–5
hopelessness 139
housing instability: LGB 95, *100*, 104
Hunter, J.: Rosario, M. and Schrimshaw, E. 104
hyperarousal 50

identity: questioning 95, *102*, 104–5
immigration 20
incarceration 9–11, 72, 82
incest 59
inclusion: LGB 92–3, **96**
income 31–2
injury 2
Institute on Trauma and Trauma-Informed Care 138–41
intergenerational trauma 6–21; ambiguous loss impacts 9–10, 20; assessment measures 13; childhood exposure to parental difficulties 14–16; coping and healing treatments 19–21; current mothering status 14–19, *17*; death impact 9; demographic characteristics 13–15, *15*; discussion 17–20; family loss risk and protective factors 7–14, 17, *17*; gender, race and ethnic differences 10–11; individual and historical 7–10; limitations and recommendations 20; study methods and results 12–17; substance use 14–16, *16*
International Association for Traumatic Stress Studies 138
International Society for the Study of Trauma and Dissociation 138
interventions: trauma-specific 4
intimate partner violence (IPV) 32, 91

Jacobs, D. 28; general theory of addictions 28, 37
Johnson, J.: and Roman, P. 117
Joint Commission on the Accreditation of Health Care Organizations (JCAHCO) 119–24
Journal of Social Work Practice in the Addictions 1–2
Jurgensen, E. 104

Keyes, K.: *et al.* 27–9
Kidd, S. 74
Knudsen, H.: Ducharme, L. and Roman, P. 117
Koenig, B.: Birkett, M. and Espelage, D. 103
Kübler-Ross, E. 19

Latina women: substance use and intergenerational trauma 6–21
Leukefeld, C.: Peden, A. and Adams, S. 47
Levene, H. 51; homogeneity test 51
lifestyle risk factors: homeless youth 67–81
loss, family 7–14, 17; and reunification projects 19–20; risk and protective factors 7–14, 17, *17*; trauma types 7–14, 17; types 14–18

marijuana 52–3, 75, 91, 104
marital status 13, 31, 50
mental health 12, 28, 32–6, 124; scores 58; status 49
mentoring 83
methamphetamines 15, 75
Meyer, I.: and Young, R. 93
mindfulness-based stress reduction 137
Mini International Neuropsychiatric Interview (MINI) 71
missing persons 9
mood disorders 29–36
mortality rate 11
mothers: Native American, Latina and White 6–21
MSM 93
Myrick, A.: and Dass-Brailsford, P. 124

Najavits, L.: and Capezza, N. 115; and Hein, D. 136; and Walsh, M. 60
naltrexone 117
National Center on Health Statistics (NCHS) 119
National Child Traumatic Stress Network (NCTSN) 137–9
National Institute on Alcohol Abuse and Alcoholism (NIAAA) 29
National Survey of Substance Abuse Treatment Services (N-SSATS, 2012) 114–15, 118, 125
Native American women 3; and cultural healing centers 19; substance use and intergenerational trauma 6–21
neglect 27–30, 72; and abuse 27–30, 33, 36–7, 72; assessment and definition 30; childhood 27–30, 33, 36–7, 72, 91; emotional 27–9; physical 30, 33, 36
neurofeedback acceptance 137
Nochajski, T.: Farrell, M. and Wolf, M. 3, 44–65
numbing 50, 68

obsessive-compulsive disorder (OCD) 49, *55*, 58
opiate dependence 45, 49, 52–3, 75
optimism 74

Padilla, Y.: *et al.* 103
panhandling 72, 82
panic disorder 44, 49; drug courts study 54–5, 60
parental difficulties: childhood exposure to 14–16
Paschall, M.: Ringwalt, C. and Flewelling, R. 83
path analysis 51, 57–8, **57**; indirect 57–8
pathological gambling disorder (PGD) 25–8, 32; and ACEs 26–8; criteria 26; negative consequences 26
pathways model/groups: gambling 28
Peden, A.: Adams, S. and Leukefeld, C. 47
Perry, B.: and Wright, E. 103–4
personality disorders 28–9
Petry, N. 30; and Steinberg, K. 27
pharmacotherapy 115
physical abuse 8, 27–32, 45, 68, 72
physical neglect 30, 33, 36
pimping 68
pornography 68
possession 50

Poteat, V.: *et al.* 105
powerlessness 10
Preferred Reporting Items for Systematic Reviews and Meta-Analyses (PRISMA) 92; guidelines 92–3
prenatal care 10
prison 11, 14; incarceration 9–11, 72, 82
programs: outpatient treatment 4, 114–26
prolonged exposure therapy (PE) 116
ProQuest Dissertations and Theses 92
prostitution 68
protective factors: and family loss risk 7–14, 17, *17*
Psychiatric Diagnostic Screening Questionnaire (PDSQ) 49–50, 53–6, *55–6*
PsychINFO 92
psychological distress 95–6, *97–8*, 103–5, 115; causes 96, 103
public health 91
PubMED 92

race 10–13, 31, 50, 116; intergenerational differences 10–11
racism 91
rage 9
rape 8, 59, 68
recovery: addiction 134–41
Resick, P. 137
resilience 2, 11–12, 69–70, 74; family 12
Resilience Scale 74
reunification projects: family 19–20
Rickman, D.: Thompson, W. and Gazel, R. 26
Ringwalt, C.: Flewelling, R. and Paschall, M. 83
risk behaviors 12; sexual 12–13
rituals 12
robbery 68
Roberts, A.: *et al.* 116
Rogers, E. 115
Roman, P.: Bride, B. and Abraham, A. 117; and Johnson, J. 117; Knudsen, H. and Ducharme, L. 117
Root Mean Square Error of Approximation (RMSEA) 57
Rosario, M.: Schrimshaw, E. and Hunter, J. 104
Ryan, C.: *et al.* 103
Sacco, P.: and Sharma, A. 3, 25–43
sanctions 54, 58–60
Sartor, C.: *et al.* 47
schizophrenia 134
Schrimshaw, E.: Hunter, J. and Rosario, M. 104
Seeking Safety (Najavits and Hein) 136, 140
self-worth 9–10
sensorimotor body processing 137
separation 28
services: welfare 10, 11, 19
services delivery, trauma 4, 115–16; eliminated programs 118; and outpatient treatment programs study 4, 114–26
sexual abuse 8, 27–32, 29–30, 68; ACE 8, 45–6; assessment 30–1; childhood 8, 28, 44–61; rates 32
sexual education 12
sexual health: gender-specific 12
sexual risk behaviors 12–13
sexual violation 2, 68; childhood 3
sexually transmitted infection (STIs) 12, 105
Shapiro, F. 137
Sharma, A.: and Sacco, P. 3, 25–43
Shields, J.: Delany, P. and Smith, K. 3, 114–29
Siegel, J.: and Williams, L. 46
Smith, K.: Shields, J. and Delany, P. 3, 114–29
Smyth, N.J. 4, 134–41; interview 134–41
social cognitive theory 83
social phobia 44, 49; drug courts study 54–5, 58, 61
social support 95, *99–100*, 103–5
social work policy 38
somatization 44; drug courts study 54–5, 60
soup kitchens 67
spare-changing 68
spirituality 12
stabilization treatments 136–40
status: education 72, 75; employment 50; marital 13, 31, 50; mothering 14–19, *17*
Steinberg, K.: and Petry, N. 27
Stevens, S.: *et al.* 3, 6–24
Stiffman, A.: Dore, P. and Elze, D. 103–4
stigma 21, 95, 104, 108
stolen goods 68
Straussner, S.L.: and Wiechelt, S.A. 1–5
stress inoculation therapy (SIT) 116

stressors 2, 8
Substance Abuse and Mental Health Services Administration (SAMHSA) 7, 91, 114–18, 124, 138; Client Outcome Measures for Discretionary Government Performance and Results Act (GPRA) 13–14; HerStory to Health program 12–21; National Center for Trauma-Informed Care (NCTIC) 135, 140
substance use disorder (SUD) 8, 18–21, 32–6, 67
SUDAAN 11 software 32
suicide 8–9, 36, 139; attempts 27, 104–5
support: social 95, *99–100*, 103–5
survival sex 68, 72, 82

theft 26, 50, 72, 82; and selling stolen goods 68
Thoma, B. 104
Thompson, S.: *et al.* 3, 66–89
Thompson, W.: Gazel, R. and Rickman, D. 26
thought-field therapy 137
training: trauma-informed care (TIC) 140–1
transience 72, 81–2
Trauma Recovery and Empowerment Model (TREM) 47
trauma types 7, 54–6, 59; definition 8; and diagnostic criteria 8; family loss 7–14, 17
trauma-informed care (TIC): and addiction recovery 134–41; emotional processing treatments 137; new developments 137; stabilization treatments 136–40; training 140–1
Traumatic Life Events Questionnaire 73
treatment: emotional processing 137; outpatient 4, 114–26; stabilization 136–40
trust 60
trustworthiness 139
Tucker-Lewis Index (TLI) 51, 57

unemployment 14, 17–18, 26
urine screens 54, 58–60
Using Trauma Theory to Design Service Systems (Harris and Fallot) 116

victimization 68, 82–5, 91, 104–5, 108; direct 73; disclosure-related 106; indirect 68, 73; LGB 95, *101–2*, 104–5, 108
violation: sexual 2, 3, 68
violence 8–11, 21; assessment 31; domestic 8, 30; interpersonal 91; intimate partner 32, 91
vocational skills education 18
vulnerability 95

Walsh, M.: and Najavits, L. 60
warrants 54, 58–60
Welch, B 51; significance test 51
welfare services 10; child 11, 19
Whitbeck, L.: *et al.* 104
White mothers 6–21
widowhood 28
Wiechalt, S.A.: and Straussner, S.L. 1–5
Williams, L.: and Siegel, J. 46
Willoughby, B.: *et al.* 103–4
Wolf, M.: Nochajski, T. and Farrell, M. 3, 44–65
women: Native American, Latina, White 3, 6–21
Wright, E.: and Perry, B. 103–4
WRMR Model Fit Index 57

Yellow Horse Brave Heart, M.: Duran, B. and Duran, E. 8
Yi, H.: Grant, B. and Harford, T. 27
yoga 137
Young, R.: and Meyer, I. 93
youth: homeless study 3, 66–85